AFRICAN-AMERICAN
Healthy

WHAT YOU NEED TO KNOW
TO PROTECT YOUR HEALTH

RICHARD W. WALKER, JR., MD

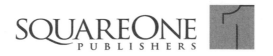

SQUAREONE
PUBLISHERS

COVER DESIGNER: Jeannie Tudor
EDITOR: Michael Weatherhead
TYPESETTER: Gary A. Rosenberg

The information and advice contained in this book are based upon the research and the personal and professional experiences of the author. They are not intended as a substitute for consulting with a health care professional. The publisher and author are not responsible for any adverse effects or consequences resulting from the use of any of the suggestions, preparations, or procedures discussed in this book. All matters pertaining to your physical health should be supervised by a health care professional. It is a sign of wisdom, not cowardice, to seek a second or third opinion.

Figure 3.1 on page 26 appears courtesy of www.wikipedia.org.
Figure 6.1 on page 60 appears courtesy of www.wikipedia.org.
Figure 6.2 on page 62 used with permission, copyright © 2011 by David G. King.

Square One Publishers
115 Herricks Road   (516) 535-2010 • (877) 900-BOOK
Garden City Park, NY 11040   www.squareonepublishers.com

Library of Congress Cataloging-in-Publication Data
Walker, Richard W.
  African-American healthy : what you need to know to protect your health /
Richard W. Walker, Jr.
    p. cm.
  ISBN 978-0-7570-0361-5
  1. Health—Popular works. 2. African Americans—Health and hygiene—Popular
works. I. Title.
  RA773.W35 2011
  613.208996073—dc22
                        2011002795

Printed in Canada

10   9   8   7   6   5   4   3   2   1

Contents

This book is dedicated to those past generations—African Americans and all others—that lacked the knowledge we have today to make the changes that would have kept themselves alive and well. In particular, it is dedicated to my parents, Richard and Ellena, who directed me as a child, giving me the wherewithal to move ahead from our menial circumstances so that I would be able to write this book. Also, to Mable Suddin, my dear mother-in-law, who died of a stroke while I was writing this book.

To the people I grew up with and all the African-American baby boomers, sorry it took me so long to get this done. To Carmen and Richard Mark, my children, and their spouses, Darrell and Rosa, this is a gift to you. I hope you'll use it to sustain your life and your family's well-being, and continue the work we all began, taking what we were given by our forefathers, and not have it interrupted by killer diseases.

To my grandchildren, Jamilla (my oldest), Samantha ("Z"), Jada Skye (the princess), Spencer (my buddy), and Leena, who'll probably take over the world, this is to you, in the hope that these issues never plague you or your families to come. I love you.

Finally, to the best friend and partner a man can have, my wife, Marvia, who has been there and endured, never wavering. Thank you for dedicating your life to me. I love you.

Foreword

As an African-American TV and radio commentator, I have heard firsthand the cries and seen the plight of so many in our community regarding the state of our health. As a single group, Black Americans top the lists of every major disease in the United States. From cancer and heart attacks to arthritis and diabetes, we have been and continue to be ravaged by these conditions. While our government officials debate the type of healthcare we need, our people are dying. Are there too few medical facilities in our neighborhoods? Is it a lack of health education on our parts? Are our lifestyles to blame? Why are we the ones to die in such great numbers from what should be treatable—and even preventable—diseases? In this tremendously important book, Dr. Richard Walker addresses all of these questions. And better yet, he offers hope by giving advice that anyone in our community can follow.

Dr. Walker is the perfect example of a concept that is deeply important to me, and that concept is community renewal. Despite his childhood health conditions, the tough environment in which he grew up, his undiagnosed dyslexia, and a system that didn't provide him with any encouragement, he worked his way up from the streets of Harlem in New York City and was able to realize his true potential. The odds were never in his favor, but he followed his dream to become a doctor, and succeeded in that goal. But for a man who has lived the life he has lived, that isn't enough.

Using the knowledge he has gained throughout his years of practice, he now wants to change the sad state of health in the African-American community. Instead of turning his back on the world in which he was raised, he is dedicating himself to making that world a better place, where parents live long enough to see their children become parents themselves, and children have the chance to grow up without feeling fated to suffer an early death due to a seemingly unavoidable chronic disease. Dr. Walker has taken his experience and combined it with today's cutting-edge science to create a book that can make a difference in so many lives.

Figures don't lie, so in this book, Dr. Walker first looks at the statistics that prove beyond a shadow of a doubt that African Americans have the highest rates in all the categories of major diseases. With that, he goes on to explain why this is happening. Not only does he carefully explain the basic causes—such as poor diet and a lack of physical activity—he goes on to look at a relatively unknown factor that may be at the center of most of these health issues. Written in clear and easy-to-understand language, Dr. Walker looks at each of these diseases and provides important information on both prevention and treatment. He also includes new suggestions based upon the latest research.

While it might take another ten years or longer for our representatives in Washington to straighten out the healthcare system in this country, most of us can begin to straighten out our own personal healthcare programs right now. Once you have read this book, you will have a choice: Either sit back and do nothing for yourself and your family, or take the information in this book and make sure that you avoid becoming another tragic statistic. I can't make that decision for you. If you've lost a family member or friend to one of these devastating illnesses, you know in your heart what you must do.

I wish you health and a lifetime of wise decisions.

Warren Ballentine, Esq.
Host of "The Warren Ballentine Show."

Introduction

I grew up in Spanish Harlem, on 115th Street between Lexington and Park Avenue, in the Johnson Housing Projects of New York City. Back then, health conditions such as hypertension, diabetes, and cancer were accepted by my community as part of the natural aging process. No one even bothered to wonder why so many black Americans were dying of these particular afflictions. Prior to his death, my own father suffered from type 2 diabetes and hypertension, which led to kidney disease, dementia, and multiple strokes. Both my maternal grandfather and grandmother also died of many of these same illnesses. But my family story was not unique. It was the same as so many other stories in the neighborhood. Black Americans were quietly being killed by their diseases and nobody was wondering why. These diseases affected not only the individual but also the family unit. A family member's illness often resulted in a loss of work hours, reduced mental alertness (resulting in fewer promotions and pay increases), and less quality time spent with the family—not to mention the greatly increased healthcare costs that prevented families from saving or investing their hard-earned money. It appeared as though type 2 diabetes, hypertension, kidney failure, stroke, heart disease, and cancer were an unavoidable part of the black experience. It was simply the way things were. Unfortunately, it's the way things still are.

The idea for this book sprang from a conversation I had with my friend Rob Martin. Rob is a pioneer of health talk radio and continues to work on the air nationwide. While discussing our family histories, we found that the health differences between Rob's Irish lineage and my own African-American one were stark. The diseases that ran through my family tree did not appear on the branches of Rob's nearly as often. This discrepancy aroused our curiosity immediately, so we compared other families we knew, both black and white, only to confirm the distinction further. Time and again, blacks seemed to get the short end of the stick when it came to general health. Most striking were the differences in longevity and cause of death. While the majority of my white friends' relatives tended to die as a result of the body's natural deterioration (what we call dying of "old age"), my black friends' family reports were littered with illnesses and rarely went beyond the basic knowledge that many of their relatives had acquired health conditions early in their lives and had died of complications from those conditions. Of course, these findings were all anecdotal, but as an African American and a doctor, my interest was piqued. Moreover, it seemed that African Americans had long ago accepted these health conditions without question, buying into the idea of a lifetime of disease management, instead of the possibility of disease prevention and reversal. Basically, the black community had come to believe that they couldn't ever expect to be as healthy as other Americans, that they could only be "African-American healthy."

Having read an enormous amount of literature over the years about the importance of vitamin D_3 in disease prevention, Rob mentioned that he had also come across studies that suggested a severe lack of this vitamin in the African-American population. We immediately wondered if this deficiency was in any way connected to the apparent tendency of African Americans towards certain illnesses. With such a depressing health disparity between blacks and whites staring me in the face, I had to wonder: Were insufficient vitamin D_3 levels making African Americans more susceptible to disease than the majority of the country? When I discovered that the answer to the question was yes, I knew I had to do something about it.

The purpose of this book is to eradicate, if possible, the predominance of disease in the black population for good. Over the course of the following chapters, you will discover the ways in which small lifestyle changes—such as adjusting your eating habits, maintaining a healthy weight, and taking vitamin D_3 and other proven supplements—can powerfully complement established medications and even prevent disease from occurring in the first place. The information found in this book aims to give you a reason to hope, to provide you with another option other than resigned acceptance of fate, which only perpetuates this silent epidemic. Ultimately, my goal is to equip African Americans—and everyone else, for that matter—with the best possible tools for illness prevention and wellness maintenance, so that we may look forward to a better future and redefine what it means to be "African-American healthy."

1

American Health in Black and White

The health disparity between black Americans and their white counterparts is wide and has been getting wider for decades. When comparisons are made between blacks and whites in relation to rates of type 2 diabetes, cardiovascular disease, kidney disease, stroke, and cancer, the results are always the same. Invariably, the incidence and severity of these illnesses are much greater in the black community. While some variance in the disease rates of different ethnicities is normal, it becomes particularly alarming when the gap is consistently and remarkably large, as it is for the black population. One look at the graph on pages 6 and 7 will show you that something is not right.[1,2,3,4]

But the health of this country need not be black and white. No matter your circumstance or skin color, the key to a long and healthy life is waiting for you to grab it. By adopting an attitude of illness prevention and recognizing the importance of diet, exercise, vitamin D_3, and other supplements, you can break free from an assumed fate of disease and early death. Once you understand the ways in which these diseases have silently infiltrated black neighborhoods all over the nation, you will realize what veritable miracles simple nutrients like vitamin D_3 can be to your health and longevity, and what huge benefits can result from simple lifestyle changes. You do not have to accept illness as an inevitable part of life anymore.

This chapter will consider the socioeconomic, cultural, genetic, and environmental aspects of the current African-American health epidemic. It will then provide an overview of the flawed concept of modern disease management and illustrate our need to move beyond it.

AFRICAN-AMERICAN HEALTH: THE SILENT EPIDEMIC

While genetics are the chief cause of the poor state of African-American health, the problem is compounded by socioeconomics, cultural beliefs, and even our modern environment. These aspects affect one another so intimately that it is impossible to understand how dire the situation has become by viewing any one of them in isolation. Over the years, they have formed a web of cause and effect that must be unraveled; otherwise, the epidemic will debilitate yet another generation.

The Socioeconomic Aspect

The truth is that healthcare costs in the United States exceed those

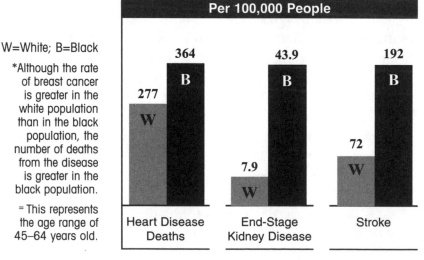

FIGURE 1.1. COMPARISON OF RATES OF DISEASE

Per 100,000 People

W=White; B=Black

*Although the rate of breast cancer is greater in the white population than in the black population, the number of deaths from the disease is greater in the black population.

= This represents the age range of 45–64 years old.

	Heart Disease Deaths	End-Stage Kidney Disease	Stroke
B	364	43.9	192
W	277	7.9	72

of almost all other major industrialized nations. Even if you are fortunate enough to have healthcare, you might go broke paying for it. The longer you live, the sicker you may get, and the more money you may spend to keep yourself alive and well. It has become a struggle to afford insurance, and a struggle to pay the co-pays and deductibles even when you do have it. Emergency Room care is available to all, regardless of income, but by the time you make it there the damage has already been done. Government-assisted medical centers can help with annual health maintenance, but the ongoing cost of medication can still be overwhelming for the underprivileged, for which rent and food for the family must often take priority over filling expensive monthly prescriptions. By the age of sixty-five, a person with a single chronic illness will spend at least $1,000 to $2,000 more per year than someone free of illness—and those costs are for people *with* Medicare.[5] The amount only gets larger as the number of diseases increases. While this reality affects everyone, it obviously hits those of lower socioeconomic status—a large number of whom are members of the black community—particularly hard.

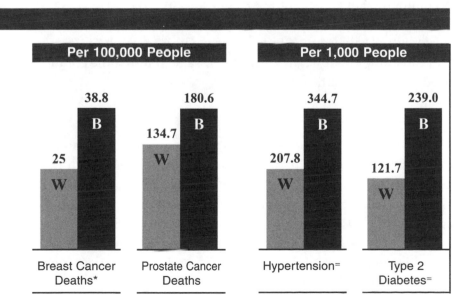

Unfortunately, healthcare in this country has made it so that an overwhelming number of African Americans—and many other Americans, in general—often put themselves in the poor house by trying to fight off illnesses with expensive treatments, only to die before their time after years of "managing" these chronic conditions. It is a heartbreaking trend. As wonderful as our doctors and hospitals are, they are still only preaching and delivering disease management, not prevention. In light of the system we have now, the best healthcare truly starts at home. As you shall soon see, by adopting simple lifestyle changes, you can not only alleviate chronic health conditions but also possibly *prevent* them from ravaging your health in the first place. Though its costs are out of control, healthcare's real problem is its blind reliance on solely drug-based therapies and its failure to promote the use of complementary non-pharmaceutical means of wellness maintenance and disease prevention. Access to care might be available, but the right *type* of care is not. The system is not making us any better. It is only maintaining the status quo. Thankfully, there is another way.

A host of conditions that commonly plague the black population can actually be avoided or significantly diminished, and all without breaking the bank. You can improve your life not only by becoming free of chronic illnesses, but also by saving the money that was formerly destined to be spent on hospital visits and drug treatments. There is an abundance of medical research out there that can guide you towards a healthy old age. But first the culture needs a change in attitude.

The Cultural Aspect

Black America has a long and justified tradition of mistrust towards medical research, dating back to around 1932, with the advent of the infamous Tuskegee experiment.

Conducted by the US Public Health Service over a forty-year span between 1932 and 1972, the Tuskegee Syphilis Study was a long-term research program that followed 399 indigent black men from Macon County, Alabama, all of whom had been diagnosed with syphilis. Instead of attempting to treat the men, the study sought to research the natural progression of the disease. This meant that even when penicillin became known as an effective cure for the illness in 1940, the study continued, denying its participants the remedy. Although there was a massive public outcry once this deplorable "research" was uncovered, the experiment nevertheless left a legacy of African-American skepticism towards the scientific community. Unfortunately, Tuskegee was just the tip of an iceberg of abuses that have been imposed on the black population, as evidenced by historical accounts of the use of slaves for medical experimentation that date as far back as 1835.[6]

Sadly, the long shadow of the Tuskegee Study continues to have a negative affect on the attitudes of black Americans. For example, a University of Pittsburgh research study reported that black parents were more apt to mistrust researchers, often believed that doctors prescribed medications as a means of experimentation, and were twice as likely as non-black parents to display skepticism towards the results of medical research in general.[7] In addition, blacks in HIV/AIDS programs have shown a reluctance to take new medications known to help control the continued mutations and growth of the HIV/AIDS virus.[8,9]

Unfortunately, this skepticism is working directly against the very real solutions that lie in wait for our community. As African Americans, we must embrace medical research, for the information it provides can be the key to our long-awaited good health. There are inexpensive ways to prevent illness, but the big pharmaceutical companies won't advertise that fact, because there simply isn't enough money in it for them. We have to find the answers for ourselves and write our own destiny as a people. The exploitation of black America must never be forgotten, but we must now open our eyes to truth when it is presented. To quote scripture: "My people are destroyed for the lack of knowledge…!" (*Hosea* 4:6)

The Genetic and Environmental Aspects

These last two aspects of African-American health are so closely intertwined that they are best understood in combination. While the socioeconomic and cultural facets of the issue definitely compound the problem, its roots can be found in our genetic make-up and the way in which our bodies react to our environment.

Research has uncovered a remarkably widespread shortage of vitamin D_3 in the bloodstream of the African-American populace. A study published in *Scientific American* revealed that approximately 97 percent of its 3,419 black Americans participants showed a deficiency in vitamin D_3. Shockingly, only 3 percent of black Americans displayed the recommended amount of this vitamin in their systems, down from 12 percent only a few decades earlier.[10] These statistics are highly troubling when you consider the importance of vitamin D_3 to human health. Evidence now shows that it plays a major role in the prevention and treatment of such illnesses as type 2 diabetes, cardiovascular disease, kidney disease, stroke, and cancer. If that list sounds familiar, take another look at the beginning of this chapter. It seems as though every condition that has been wreaking havoc on the black community can be directly connected to low levels of vitamin D_3 in the body, from which almost the entire black population suffers. To understand how one segment of the population could have become so thoroughly deficient in this vitamin, we must first learn a little more about it.

Vitamin D_3 is known as the "sunshine vitamin" because sunlight is required for the body to manufacture it. This rule applies to everybody on the planet, not just blacks and other dark-skinned racial groups. As you probably know from countless sunscreen commercials, the body is bombarded on a daily basis by UV (short for ultraviolet) rays from the sun. While too much UV light exposure can be harmful to our health, a certain amount is necessary for our systems to function properly. The absorption by the skin of one particular kind of UV light, called UVB rays, promotes the production of vitamin D_3 in the body. As an African American, the dark pigmentation of your skin causes less of these UVB rays to be absorbed. Unfortunately, it seems as though genetics are conspiring against dark-complexioned people. Historically speaking, though, our skin color has been advantageous, in that it protected us from harmful UV damage. During the days when our ancestors lived near the equator and worked predominantly out-doors in the oppressive sun, our genetics worked to our benefit. Our dark skin produced sufficient levels of vitamin D_3 from the abundance of sunlight while simultaneously safeguarding us from the ill-effects of too much ultraviolet light. These days our every-day environment is much different. Most of our time is spent working indoors, and even a good portion of our weekend takes place inside the home. And unlike our ancestors, many of us now live far from the equator, in cold climates that offer less vitamin D_3-producing sunlight for a large portion of the year.

For a race of people that requires generous amounts of sun-light in order to function optimally, modernity has quietly creat-ed a big problem. The combination of our genetics and our contemporary lives is proving deadly. Thankfully, with a drug store in almost every town of the country, the solution to decades of insufficient vitamin D_3 levels couldn't be closer. Vitamin sup-plements are available and relatively inexpensive. By looking at the compelling research on vitamin D_3 and its role in disease pre-vention, we as black Americans can now begin to avoid illnesses once considered inevitable. But to permanently close the unnec-essary racial health gap to which we've grown tragically accus-tomed, we need to move beyond the typically prescribed routines of "disease management."

DISEASE MANAGEMENT

Current medical training is designed around the early adoption of pharmaceutical treatments for most health problems. While tradi-tional medications certainly have their place, doctors too often address only the symptoms of a condition rather than its root cause, neglecting the steps that can be taken to prevent it. It seems that we have a *disease* system rather than a *health* system. The mod-ern concept of "disease management" hinders the health progress not only of black Americans but of all Americans. Sicknesses that can and should be remedied by simple lifestyle modifications, such as vitamin D_3 supplementation and proper nutrition, are being prolonged and "managed" by expensive drugs that frequently lead to other, more powerful expensive drugs.

Let's take, as an example, the disease of type 2 diabetes, which we will discuss in greater detail in Chapter 7. Type 2 diabetes often occurs when obesity, stress, and lack of exercise combine to increase the body's insulin level, which, over time, can cause cell membranes to lose their sensitivity to its effect. This result, in turn, causes an unhealthy rise in the body's blood sugar. Traditional disease management of type 2 diabetes aims to control the elevation of the patient's blood sugar by artificially inhibiting the production and release of glucose from the liver or, in more severe cases, supplying the body with more insulin for its desensitized cells. With a few exceptions in the medical community, there is little mention of restoring the cells' response mechanisms by lowering the overall production of insulin back to normal levels through nutrition and exercise, which would thereby allow for better blood sugar control naturally. One method treats the source of the illness, while the other manages only its symptoms. Instead of addressing the causes of disease, we are asked to subscribe to a routine of medications that are the equivalent of an extremely costly band-aid. Disease management is designed to get you by, not to get you healthy. It's no wonder we find it so difficult to improve our situation. As you will see throughout this book, this disease—as well as those illnesses we mentioned previously—can be brought under control and even eradicated by simple changes in everyday conduct. You need not follow the road to nowhere any longer. You just have to stop thinking only in terms of disease management and start thinking in terms of wellness maintenance and illness prevention.

As you go through the next chapters, you'll begin to see why the accepted forms of disease management are no longer a sufficient answer to *any* of the illnesses affecting the black community. Instead of treating mere symptoms, we need to tackle our problems at their source. Only then will we reduce the occurrence of these silent killers, minimize the amount of income spent on treatments, and increase the quality and length of our lives.

FAMILY HISTORY, NOT DESTINY

Family history is not the same as genetic predisposition. At the moment, when doctors speak of genetic illness, they are referring to conditions the expression of which little can be done to prevent or alter. For example, type 1 diabetes is a genetic disease and therefore beyond your control to avoid. It is not caused or alleviated by lifestyle. Lifestyle can certainly make the disease worse, but it does not set it in motion. In contrast, type 2 diabetes *can* be caused by lifestyle choices, and also dramatically improved by them. This type of illness is due to many things other than genes, such as environment and cultural habits, both of which we can change. Simply because a disease such as type 2 diabetes seems to run in your family does not mean that you are destined to be stricken with it yourself. Once you realize that disease can sometimes be brought on by lifestyle choices, those lifestyle choices can be modified or even changed outright. Your future does not have to include sickness. But to step outside of your family history of disease, you must first summon the will to change your habits and acquire the knowledge required to make that change. By reading this book, you are already on your way.

CONCLUSION

As you have now seen, poor health is a multi-faceted and deeply rooted problem in the black community. It is so deeply rooted, in fact, that it includes our very genetics as a cause. While research suggests that vitamin D_3 might reverse or even prevent all sorts of diseases—including the very afflictions that have been cutting the black community off at its knees for so long—our contemporary lifestyles prevent us from getting the amount of sunlight required by our dark-skinned bodies to produce it sufficiently. As a result, we are becoming more and more deficient in this important biological tool and, in turn, getting sicker than other racial groups. And as long as the medical establishment continues to preach a system of typical disease management and not prevention, we will continue on the path to early death.

Knowledge truly is power. In this book you will find all the information required to begin a health revolution. By harnessing the disease-fighting properties of vitamin D_3, adjusting your diet, and maintaining a normal weight, you can improve the overall quality of your life and help reclaim the future of your community. It is time to turn the page.

2

Understanding and Slowing the Aging Process

Premature illness and death are a hallmark of black American life, and have been for so long that, unfortunately, the black community has come to accept aging as a series of prolonged and inescapable battles against a variety of health conditions. While the body's ideal state does deteriorate as it gets older, you need not assume a life filled with disease. Regardless of ethnicity, you can remain healthy and active throughout your later years. Now that you have learned about the specific plight of African-American health and its tightly interwoven causes and effects, I would like to address the concept of aging in general. In doing so, we will be able to better understand the normal changes that occur in the human body as it grows older and reevaluate the inevitability of illness as a natural part of the process.

THE VICIOUS CIRCLE

When I tell you that cell deterioration is an ordinary part of the course of aging and that disease-promoting molecules are naturally produced by your body every single day, you might want to throw your hands up in frustration and give up trying to age healthily. The longer you live, the more damage your system encounters, thereby becoming less effective at fighting further damage, thereby incurring more damage, and so on. But the simple fact that these processes are unavoidable does not mean that you cannot substantially slow the aging process and maintain your health for years to come. Watching what you eat, maintaining a proper vitamin intake, and managing your enzyme and hormone levels are all ways in which you can lessen the effects of aging and stave off many of the diseases that have come to accompany growing older.

Cell Deterioration

Although there are many technical theories of aging, the truth is no one really knows exactly why it occurs. In generalized terms, the aging process is the natural deterioration of cellular function. As cells grow older, their ability to function diminishes. This decline in capability—called *senescence*—has significant effects on the human body. While scientists are hard at work trying to understand and slow the aging process, for now we all still have to face this stage of life.

To illustrate the biological transformations associated with aging, I will use the example of liver cells, also called *hepatocytes*. One of the most important operations of the liver is its role in the detoxification of our blood. It performs the first phase of this job through the production of a host of enzymes called *cytochromes P450*, or P450. These enzymes are responsible for metabolizing that which our body naturally produces (called *endogenous substances*) as well as that which the body takes in from its environment, such as medications, food, water, air, and anything absorbed through the skin (called *exogenous substances*). Through the process of metabolism, the chemical compounds inherent to each substance are broken down and converted into simpler molecules, which are then either utilized by the body or eliminated from it. For those molecules that require elimination, P450 enzymes must first convert them from fat-soluble particles into water-soluble particles, so that they can then be excreted from the body through sweat, stool, urine, and exhalation, thus detoxifying the body.

Unfortunately, as your liver ages, the effectiveness of its enzymes begins to decrease. Without properly functioning P450 enzymes, the process of elimination breaks down and toxins begin to accumulate in your system. The more toxins remaining in your body, the quicker the deterioration of your body's cells will be. Thus begins a relentless process of degeneration. Cells grow old and lose their efficacy, which leads to a buildup of toxins in your body, which leads to further deterioration of cells. It is a vicious circle that can quickly lead to disease unless something is done to slow it down.

Keep in mind that the preceding example focuses on just one organ system and one set of cells in that organ. Now imagine this process occurring throughout all the organ systems of your body simultaneously, without anything being done to reduce its consequences. If the deterioration of cells goes without interruption, your worst fears about aging will be proven correct. Disease will inexorably follow the steady march of declining cellular function, much as it does from the unchecked proliferation of free radicals, which I will now discuss.

Free Radicals

Each cell of your body is made up of molecules, which themselves consist of two or more atoms that have formed a chemical bond. Contained in each atom is a nucleus surrounded by pairs of electrons. When one of these pairs loses an electron, the atom becomes unstable. In this state, it seeks to stabilize itself by bouncing around randomly in search of another electron to complete its unbalanced pair, eventually stealing one from a neighboring molecule or atom. This causes a chain reaction, as the neighboring molecule or atom now possesses an unpaired electron itself and sets off to affect the first compound *it* finds. Free to attack and rob from any cell component it wishes, these electron thieves are appropriately called *free radicals* and can be profoundly destructive to your system. Left unchecked, they can quickly damage cells, thus accelerating the aging process and leading to disease.

Unfortunately, free radicals are a perfectly normal by-product of metabolism. In fact, the very air you breathe plays a role in the production of one of the most destructive free radicals, named the *reactive oxygen species,* or ROS. Your *mitochondria,* which are the energy factories of every cell, use oxygen molecules to metabolize sugars and fats into the energy you use every day, leaving behind unbalanced oxygen-centered atoms as a result. While your body does release compounds on its own to neutralize these free radicals, it cannot eliminate them all. Over time, they slowly accumulate, causing what is called *oxidative stress.* The more oxidative stress you endure, the quicker your body will age, the more likely you will be to acquire diseases, and the less able your cells will be to prevent more free radicals from forming.

HOW TO KEEP YOUR GOLDEN YEARS GOLDEN

Just because things like free radicals and cell deterioration occur naturally does not mean that you have to take them lying down. Taking certain vitamins, eating particular foods, and maintaining your enzyme and hormone levels can help your body eliminate free radicals and impede cell death. This, in turn, can delay and decrease the destructive effects of aging, reduce the incidence of illness, and enable you to grow old gracefully, whatever your racial background.

Antioxidants and Hormones

While your system regularly produces protective molecules called *antioxidants* to fight off oxidative stress, your body does not generally produce sufficient antioxidants to defend against every free radical. You can, however, increase the supply of antioxidants in your body through diet and vitamin supplementation. Citrus fruits, green vegetables, nuts, and legumes all contain a wide variety of different antioxidants, including vitamins A, C, and E. In contrast to black and oolong teas, green tea maintains a high level of the powerful antioxidant *epigallocatechin gallate,* or EGCG, due to its leaves being steamed instead of fermented. Although red wine contains it to a greater degree, the antioxidant *resveratrol* is found in both red and white wine. And those of you with a sweet tooth will be thrilled to hear that dark chocolate provides a significant amount of antioxidants called *flavonoids*, though these particular compounds are removed from milk chocolate because of their bitter taste.

While I ultimately recommend getting your antioxidants from real food sources, I do realize that sometimes life gets in the way of a proper meal. A daily multivitamin can be helpful to fill in the gaps in your diet.

A class of enzymes called the *superoxide dismutase,* or SOD, is another important antioxidant. These enzymes are naturally produced by your body to reduce the most destructive free radicals, known as the reactive oxygen species, and help slow the vicious circle of aging. But when cells have been damaged over the years and no longer generate SOD enzymes in sufficient amounts, it may be time to turn to medical science, which has made it possible to take them orally. I recommend a dosage of 150 mg per day, but your doctor may suggest a slightly different amount for your individual needs.

My final suggestion to manage aging effectively and ward off its adverse effects involves the growing field of medicine that deals with hormone restoration. Hormones are the body's chemical messengers. The word *hormone* is derived from the ancient Greek word *hormao,* which literally means "I set in motion," and this is exactly what hormones do—they set chemical reactions in motion within our bodies, causing cells to perform the various functions for which they are responsible. Some hormones encourage cellular activity, some suppress it, and some even turn other hormones on or off. You may have heard of hormones such as *testosterone*—the predominant hormone in men—and *estrogen* and *progesterone*—the predominant hormones in women—but there are actually about sixty different hormones at work in the human body. Even the focus of this book, vitamin D_3, itself acts as a hormone once it is synthesized by your liver or kidneys, regulating the concentration of calcium and phosphate in your bloodstream, encouraging healthy bone production, and stimulating the creation of enzymes that fight off free radicals.[1]

As you age, however, hormone production diminishes, resulting in many of the symptoms associated with becoming a senior citizen. In men, this decrease in production begins at approximately age thirty and progresses slowly. In women, it starts sometime around the age of forty-five, but progresses more rapidly. Loss of muscle and muscle definition, memory loss, brain fog, uncontrolled weight gain, fatigue, mood swings, and hot flashes are all tied to decreasing hormone manufacture. For a long time, these problems were generally dismissed as inevitable, with the patient being sent home with a diagnosis of "You're just getting old!" Fortunately, this is no longer the case. Doctors can now identify which hormones require restoration and correct their decline by providing hormone replacement treatments.[2] Dosage is based on your symptoms, height, weight, and family history of cancer. While I recommend bioidentical hormones over synthetic hormones, therapy of either kind has its risks and potential side effects, so it is important to discuss all the pros and cons of any treatment you may be considering with your doctor before beginning any hormone regimen. New information is being uncovered every day in this field.

CONCLUSION

By understanding the normal process of aging, we can conclude that the killer diseases so commonly seen in the elderly population do not have to be its natural consequence. While you cannot stop your cells from growing older, you can easily take steps to decrease the speed with which their decreased functionality wreaks havoc on your system. Simply following a balanced diet that is rich in vegetables and fruits can give you the vitamins and antioxidants your body requires to slow cell death and reduce the occurrence of disease. When that is not enough, there are multivitamins and other supplements to help you conserve your energy and well-being.

Though these recommendations apply to everyone, they are particularly important to African-Americans, for whom socioeconomic and cultural considerations have made things like eating right and getting the proper amount of vitamins and antioxidants so difficult. Couple that fact with our biological deficiency of one of the most important safeguards against cell deterioration, vitamin D_3, and you will recognize just how crucial the information found in this book is to the health of the black community. The only true killer we face is ignorance.

3

Vitamin D₃

As you already know, the primary focus of this book is vitamin D_3, a nutrient that has been found to be beneficial in more ways than you may have thought possible. But exactly what is vitamin D_3, and why aren't most people getting enough of it? More importantly, what can vitamin D_3 do for you as you seek greater health? This chapter will answer these questions and more so that you fully appreciate how D_3 combats disease and supports a long and healthy life.

WHAT ARE VITAMINS?

Like other essential nutrients such as carbohydrates, proteins, and fats, vitamins are chemical compounds that cannot be synthesized by the body in sufficient amounts to maintain proper health. As a result, they must be obtained from the environment. Unlike carbohydrates, proteins, and fats, however, vitamins are required only in very small amounts and are therefore categorized as *micronutrients*—though they certainly play a large role in many biochemical functions throughout the body. For example, vitamin A helps control cell and tissue growth, while vitamin D regulates the concentration of calcium and phosphate in the bloodstream. Vitamins C and E act as antioxidants, protecting cells by scavenging free radicals.[1] Vitamin B_7 helps break down fats and carbohydrates, and vitamin B₉ aids in the production of new cells. While you do not need to know the minute details of each vitamin's role, you should understand that the processes made possible by these nutrients are critical to your survival.[2]

Vitamins are classified into two separate groups according to the way in which they are dissolved in your system. Vitamins that are dissolved in lipids, or fats, are called *fat-soluble* vitamins. This category includes vitamins A, D, E, and K. Any surplus of fat-soluble vitamins gets stored in the liver and can be used by the body when needed. Vitamins that dissolve in water are called *water-soluble* vitamins. This category includes vitamin C and the B family of vitamins. Unlike their fat-soluble counterparts, these water-soluble vitamins are easily eliminated through urination and therefore must be replenished much more regularly.

While food has been a good source of vitamins for countless years, variations in the food supply due to famine, drought, geographic location, farming techniques, and socioeconomic status have negatively affected the health of many people. Thankfully, vitamin supplements now allow for the support of general health and the treatment of deficiency-related disorders.[3]

WHAT IS VITAMIN D₃?

Vitamin D was first discovered in 1919 by Sir Edward Mellanby, an English physician and professor who had been researching the cause of rickets, a debilitating childhood bone disease. By experimenting with the diets of dogs—and also inadvertently depriving them of vitamin D-producing sunlight—he was able to link the origin of the illness with the absence of a trace component in the diet. Shortly thereafter, American biochemist E.V. McCollum identified the missing trace component as vitamin D. Since then, there has been an ever-growing amount of information written about this vital substance.

Vitamin D comes from the cholesterol in your body's cells and is fat-soluble. As most of the body's tissues have fat in them, it is easily absorbed. Vitamin D is not only a vitamin but also a *pro-*

hormone, which means it is a precursor to a hormone. Hormones are chemicals in the body that stimulate and repress the functions of other cells. In other words, they tell cells what to do and what not to do. Once vitamin D gets converted by the skin, liver, or kidneys, it takes on hormone-like properties, essentially becoming a hormone itself. Five forms of vitamin D exist, though only two of them are relevant to humans. These two forms are vitamin D_2 (called *ergocalciferol*) and vitamin D_3 (called *cholecalciferol*). While there is some debate regarding which form is best to take as a supplement, most physicians now recommend D_3 because it has proven to be the more bioactive of the two, which simply means that it does what it is supposed to do more effectively. Before buying vitamin supplements, it is always a good idea to research which form of each nutrient is the most bioactive. By choosing a brand that features the most bioactive form of each vitamin, you will know that you're getting the full benefits of supplementation. Because it is so important to your health, I want you to know that the bioactivity of vitamin D_3 is absolutely crucial to the quality and length of your life.

The essence of vitamin D_3's potential health benefits still has not reached the general population of the United States. Most people know more about the medications they see on television, which have high costs and high risks, than what they do about this low-cost, low-risk miracle nutrient. While this is a shame for everyone in the country, it is especially terrible for African Americans, who are the most deficient in vitamin D_3.

HOW IS VITAMIN D₃ MADE?

Your skin is made up of two layers: the outer, thinner layer called the *epidermis,* and the inner, deeper layer called the *dermis.* From outermost to innermost, the epidermis consists of five layers called the *stratum corneum,* the *stratum lucidum,* the *stratum granulosum,* the *stratum spinosum,* and the *stratum basale.* (See Figure 3.1.) The dermis is composed largely of connective tissue, which literally holds everything together. When ultraviolet radiation (also

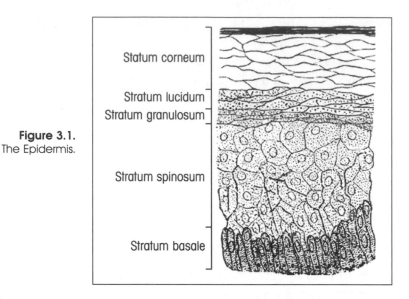

Statum corneum

Stratum lucidum
Stratum granulosum

Figure 3.1.
The Epidermis.

Stratum spinosum

Stratum basale

called UV radiation) from sunlight reaches the stratum spinosum and stratum basale layers of the skin—the deepest layers of the epidermis—it creates a photochemical reaction that converts a molecule called *7-dehydrocholestrerol* into Vitamin D_3.[4] The three most important factors in vitamin D_3 production are the type of UV radiation to which you are exposed, your amount of exposure to this UV radiation, and the concentration of a molecular compound called *melanin* in your skin.[5]

The photochemical reaction responsible for the creation of vitamin D_3 is dependent upon a type of UV radiation called UVB rays. (See the inset on page 27.) UVB light is the only kind of sunlight able to penetrate the skin far enough to set the reaction in motion. The more time spent in the sun, the more UVB rays are able to reach your deepest epidermal layers, and thus the more vitamin D_3 will be manufactured. But because UVB exposure is determined by the position of the sun in the sky, it fluctuates all too easily. It varies according to the time of day, the time of year, and even where you live.

UVB light is strongest between 11:00 AM and 2:00 PM, when the sun is at its highest point in the sky. Conversely, when the sun is too low, most UVB radiation is absorbed by the atmosphere before reaching your body. UVB intensity is also affected considerably by the time of year and your place of residence. If you live anywhere above the 37° latitude (which would be anywhere above San Jose, California), your exposure to vitamin D-producing radiation is almost non-existent between the months of November and February due to your location in relation to the sun. This should come as a revelation to black Americans who live in the northern region of the country, as we require even more UVB light to synthesize vitamin D₃ than our light-skinned neighbors. It might also explain why Africans who have immigrated to less sunny, northern parts of the world such as Sweden and Norway are more vitamin-D₃ deficient than their former countrymen who live closer to the equator.

This last fact brings us to the final factor in vitamin D₃ creation: your body's concentration of melanin. Melanin is a compound that filters ultraviolet light from the stratum spinosum and stratum basale of your skin. This fact is extremely important for African Americans, whose skin is dark as a result of a high concentration of melanin. In short, the more melanin in your body, the darker your skin will be, and the greater amount of UVB exposure

What Is UVB Light?

Essentially, light is electromagnetic radiation that travels in wave-shaped patterns. The distance between each wave peak in a pattern is aptly called the wavelength, which is calculated in fractions of a meter. Measured in nanometers, or 10 to the power of minus 9 meters, UV light has extremely short wavelengths that make it invisible to the human eye. The spectrum of UV light ranges from 10 to 400 nm, with vitamin D3-producing UVB rays occurring at a wavelength between 280-320 nm. In fact, for optimal vitamin D3 synthesis to occur, an even narrower band of UVB wavelength between 295-300 nm is needed, with the absolute ideal wavelength being exactly 297 nm. This narrower UVB band of light is referred to as deep ultraviolet light, or DUV.

will be required to synthesize vitamin D_3. As our modern lifestyles continue to take us out of the sunlight, it is easy to see why dark-complexioned people all over the country are becoming more and more deficient in this disease-fighting substance.

OTHER SOURCES OF VITAMIN D_3

While nothing produces vitamin D_3 quite like sunshine, there are other ways to get the nutrient. Natural food sources of vitamin D_3 include fish such as salmon, tuna, and eel; as well as cod liver oil. There are also small amounts of the vitamin in cheese and egg yolks. Though some types of mushrooms contain vitamin D, it is in the less bioactive form of vitamin D_2, which makes them the least ideal food source. Over the past few decades, the United States government has allowed other foods to be fortified with vitamin D, including milk, orange juice, and breakfast cereal. Finally, because food is not always a sufficient source of the nutrient, supplements can be added to your diet in an effort to maintain proper D_3 levels.

HOW DOES VITAMIN D_3 WORK?

Once vitamin D_3 is produced via UVB exposure from the sun, consumed in food, or absorbed through supplements, it is then converted by the liver and kidneys into its bioactive form, called *1,25-dihydroxyvitamin D_3*.[6] Once converted, this hormone-like form of vitamin D_3 is transported to the various cells of your body, attaching to a receptor in the nucleus of each cell. After reaching its destination, it then turns the genes of that cell on or off. In other words, it either causes or prevents the cell from doing something in your body.

WHAT CAN VITAMIN D_3 DO FOR YOU?

While all vitamins are important, vitamin D_3 seems to be the most exciting of all, as it seems that there is no end to the positive effects it can have on human physiology. Depending on the cell to which it is delivered, vitamin D_3 can affect a wide range of bodily functions, such as insulin secretion and sensitivity, calcium absorption, and your immune system's ability to fight cancers and other foreign invaders such as viruses. The following discussions each give a brief explanation of the connection between vitamin D_3 and good health. Later chapters will provide further details to give you a more complete picture of the powerful role this nutrient can play in your well-being.

Bacterial, Viral, Fungal, and Parasitic Infection

It has been proven that Vitamin D_3 stimulates the genes in your immune system that are responsible for the production of molecules called *antimicrobial peptides.* Antimicrobial peptides act as natural antibiotics in the body, protecting it against viral, bacterial, fungal, and parasitic infections. By raising the amount of vitamin D_3 in your body, you also increase the number of these infection-fighting molecules. For example, at the height of the tuberculosis outbreaks of the 1940s and '50s, doctors would place patients in sunlight as much as possible, thus elevating their levels of vitamin D_3. Those who got lots of sunlight proved less susceptible to the disease than those who did not, and recovered quicker if they had already contracted it.

Bone Density

Most people who know about vitamin D_3 are mainly familiar with its effect on bones. It is commonly used in conjunction with calcium supplementation to ensure absorption of the bone-strengthening mineral. By aiding calcium in its function, vitamin D_3 prevents bone deterioration and fracture due to osteopenia and osteoporosis, two conditions marked by low bone mineral density.

Cancer

It is now clear that an increased level of vitamin D_3 is connected to a reduction of at least seventeen different types of cancer, including skin, breast, and prostate cancer. In fact, studies have suggested that vitamin D_3 deficiency may be a leading *cause* of such disorders.[7]

Depression

Seasonal affective disorder refers to depression that commonly occurs during the winter months, when vitamin D-producing sunlight is at its least potent. In a study that included 1,282 subjects, researchers at the University of Amsterdam reported that those people with the lowest levels of vitamin D_3 also had the highest rates of depression.[8]

Type 2 Diabetes

Most people are aware that rates of type 2 diabetes are at epidemic proportions around the world. This form of diabetes—also called *adult-onset diabetes* because of the typical age at which it occurs—is characterized by a decrease in the body's production of insulin or a reduction of the body's sensitivity to it, both of which cause an inability to maintain proper blood sugar levels. A direct relationship has been shown between low levels of vitamin D_3 and a higher incidence of diabetes, while increases in vitamin D_3 appear to improve sensitivity to insulin.[9]

Disease in Children

Low levels of vitamin D_3 in children are associated with an increase in heart disease and the childhood bone disease rickets. In fact, the risk of both illnesses is even higher for children of color, who are typically more deficient in the nutrient than their light-skinned friends.[10]

Hypertension and Heart Disease

Like depression, an increase in cases of hypertension (also known as high blood pressure) during the winter months suggests a connection with decreased levels of vitamin D_3-producing sunshine. Approximately 50 percent of all cases of high blood pressure in

African Americans and other dark-skinned people are connected to insufficient amounts of vitamin D_3 in the body.[11] Left untreated, hypertension can easily lead to a hardening of the arteries, also called *atherosclerosis*, which can lead to a heart attack. Numerous studies have shown that the incidence of heart attacks due to atherosclerosis increases dramatically in individuals that have a vitamin D_3 deficiency.[12]

Life Span

White blood cells, also called *leukocytes,* help protect your body from foreign invaders and illness. Leukocytes are themselves protected by a part of the cell called the *telomere.* A telomere can best be illustrated by thinking of a shoelace. At the end of a shoelace is a hard piece of plastic that keeps the string from unraveling. Consider that piece of plastic wrapped around the string as the telomere wrapped around a piece of DNA. The length of a telomere is directly related to the life span of your cells and thus to *your* life span. The longer the telomere, the greater the life span of that cell. Studies now show that vitamin D_3 can help keep these protective structures long and strong.[13]

CONCLUSION

The illnesses listed above are just a few of the conditions that can be addressed by the untapped potential of vitamin D_3. I have no doubt that you now understand just how important adequate levels of this nutrient are, especially to African Americans, whose dark skin makes the production of vitamin D_3 a more difficult task. Vitamin D_3 deficiency can negatively affect nearly every aspect of your life if you let it persist. In addition, it can affect the lives of the people closest to you, namely your children, your siblings, your parents, and your best friends. Throughout the following chapters, you will discover how vitamin D_3 can help you avoid a range of health conditions.

4

Hypertension

Hypertension, commonly known as high blood pressure, is a condition of the cardiovascular system. The cardiovascular system is made up of the heart and blood vessels, which circulate blood throughout the body. Although hypertension is only one of the many conditions that can affect your cardiovascular system, it deserves particularly close attention, as it usually leads to much deadlier forms of cardiovascular disease. Unfortunately, approximately 1.6 billion people worldwide suffer from hypertension. It is often called the "silent killer" because of the way in which it quietly and slowly damages your body, producing few, if any, symptoms until it is too late. If left unchecked, hypertension can result in illnesses that prove far more dangerous and difficult to treat. It was the root cause of many of the health conditions that killed my father, including kidney disease, stroke, and eventually heart failure.

While high blood pressure is undoubtedly a problem for individuals of every color and ethnicity, it has become a signature condition of the black community over the last few decades, occurring three to five times as often in black Americans than it does in white Americans. As a result, there are much higher rates of stroke, kidney failure, and congestive heart failure in the black population than in the white population. Adding to the severity of these statistics is the fact that doctors are now starting to see high blood pressure not only in black adults but also in black adolescents. Because many healthcare providers still do not recognize the possibility of such an early onset of hypertension, they do not test for it. High blood pressure in young people, therefore, could be even more widespread than we know. It is a scary thought. In light of this information, it is no wonder that the disease rates of African Americans remain so high.[1]

This chapter will provide you with a better understanding of hypertension, the factors that contribute to its development, and the ways in which it can be overcome. In doing so, you will be taking a vitally important step towards avoiding the killer diseases that too frequently follow a diagnosis of hypertension.

WHAT IS HYPERTENSION?

The heart is basically a pump that circulates the blood in your body. Blood leaves the heart through vessels called *arteries*, is carried to and from tissues through vessels called *capillaries*, and returns to the heart through vessels called *veins.* As blood gets pumped into the arteries, it exerts pressure on the walls of those blood vessels. This force is appropriately called *blood pressure.* Hypertension is an elevation of that pressure, which is why it is also referred to simply as high blood pressure. If left untreated, hypertension can result in life-threatening physiological damage, as it is one of the major risk factors for atherosclerosis. Atherosclerosis, as you know from Chapter 3, is a hardening of the arteries due to a buildup of plaque along the walls of the blood vessels. As the walls of your arteries thicken with plaque, you become more and more prone to heart attacks and stroke, as it becomes increasingly difficult for your heart to move blood throughout your body. For example, with every increase of 7 points in diastolic blood pressure above 90 mmHg, your likelihood of a heart attack also increases by 27 percent, while your chance of having a stroke increases by 42 percent.[2] (To learn about diastolic blood pressure, see the inset "How High Is High Blood Pressure?," on page 35.)

How High Is High Blood Pressure?

Blood pressure is represented by a pair of numbers. The first number is systolic pressure, which refers to the force exerted by your blood every time your heart beats, pushing your blood throughout your body. The second number is diastolic pressure, which refers to the pressure placed on your blood vessels while your heart rests between beats. Blood pressure readings are measured in millimeters of mercury, or mmHG, which is the height a column of mercury reaches under the pressure created by your blood.

A normal blood pressure reading is approximately 120 over 80 mmHG, or 120/80. Readings between 130/80 and 139/89 are considered prehypertension, while any reading over 140/90 is considered hypertension. An official diagnosis of hypertension (high blood pressure) is made when two or more blood pressure readings average 140/90 or above over a seventy-two-hour period.

Because of the seriousness of high blood pressure, the benefits of traditional medications to treat hypertension usually outweigh their risks. These pharmaceutical therapies, however, too often lead to the mindset of typical disease management, the problems of which I discussed in Chapter 1. Often these medications do not fully resolve hypertension or the damage associated with it. But what if vitamin D_3 and other alternative treatments could improve and even prevent the need for these commonly used therapies? The answer to this question could save your life.

WHAT CAUSES HYPERTENSION?

While no clear-cut cause of high blood pressure has been determined, research has identified a handful of factors that contribute to the problem. These factors include vitamin D_3 deficiency and type 2 diabetes, as well as lifestyle considerations such as stress, lack of exercise, high salt intake, and smoking. Some are easier to fix than others, but they must all be addressed and understood.

Vitamin D₃ Deficiency and the Renin-Angiotensin-Aldosterone System

The *renin-angiotensin-aldosterone system,* or RAAS, is a hormone system that regulates blood pressure and balances water levels in the body. Renin is an enzyme that stimulates the production of angiotensin, a protein. This protein causes blood vessels to constrict, thus raising blood pressure. Angiotensin then stimulates the production of the hormone aldosterone, which causes the body to reabsorb more water and sodium into the blood. This elevation in fluid, in turn, increases blood pressure even further. When it is functioning properly, the RAAS becomes active in response to drops in blood pressure. Unfortunately, it can also be set in motion by abnormally high levels of renin, which some studies suggest could be the result of a vitamin D_3 deficiency.

Because vitamin D_3 prevents the overproduction of renin, any deficiency in this nutrient inevitably leads to an increased amount of renin in the body and, eventually, hypertension.[3] According to a report in *The Journal of Hypertension,* at least 50 percent of all cases of hypertension in dark-skinned Americans can be linked to low levels of vitamin D_3.[4] This is a truly staggering statistic that can be easily improved.

Salt

Your body requires a small amount of salt every day to function properly. Too much salt, however, can be a health risk. When your body has more salt than your kidneys can pass into your urine, the excess accumulates in your bloodstream. This elevation in salt levels causes your body to retain water, drawing it into your blood in an effort to bring itself back into balance. The retained water increases the volume of blood in your system, which raises your blood pressure.

While you only need about 500 mg of salt daily for good health, most people get more than ten times that amount. If you suffer from high blood pressure, you would benefit from keeping your daily salt intake to a maximum of 1,500 mg.

Sedentary Lifestyle

Research shows that a sedentary lifestyle contributes to an elevation in blood pressure. A study of 13,748 people revealed an increase in inflammation—the first step in high blood pressure—in those who did not exercise and a decrease in inflammation in those who did.[5] In addition, patients who have had or are at risk of having a heart attack invariably show great improvements once they adopt a regular exercise regimen.[6] Simply put, exercise is known to reduce blood pressure in people with hypertension as well as in those who have normal blood pressure. Exercise not only brings down your blood pressure, it also improves other health problems, including obesity and insulin resistance, which are themselves contributors to hypertension.[7]

Smoking

Although most people associate smoking with lung cancer, the nasty habit also substantially increases your risk of developing high blood pressure. Cigarette smoke causes blood vessels to spasm; increases LDL, or "bad," cholesterol; lowers HDL, or "good," cholesterol; results in inflammation of the endolethium; and promotes blood clots. If that weren't enough to make you quit lighting up, smoking also creates lots of free radicals and negates the positive effects of vitamin D_3 in the body. Needless to say, the numerous biological consequences of smoking are directly associated with heart disease and early death.

Stress

Stress results in the production of a hormone called *cortisol*. Cortisol is nicknamed the "death hormone" for its ability to increase blood pressure, which can slowly result in deadly heart attacks and strokes. Stress is a particular concern for African Americans, many of whom unknowingly suffer from a silent coping mechanism known as *John Henryism*, which increases blood pressure.[8]

The term John Henryism comes from the African-American folklore hero John Henry, who worked himself to death trying to compete with a steam-powered machine. It refers to a method of dealing with stress in which a high degree of effort is extended against psychological stressors over a prolonged period of time. It is marked by a personality that is preoccupied with success, especially in unfamiliar environments in which there is very little support. These traits are directly linked to hypertension and disease.

Although there is debate regarding the causes of John Henryism, some in the medical field have suggested a genetic predisposition for the condition in African Americans. Whether or not this is the case, environmental factors such as nutrition can have an affect on the expression of that coping style, which is why it is so important to consider all avenues of treatment for hypertension, not just traditional medications.[9] A few lifestyle changes, such as a healthful diet and exercise, can have a tremendous impact on the way in which you handle stress.

Type 2 Diabetes

Due to its tendency to harden arteries, type 2 diabetes is known to cause high blood pressure. According to the American Diabetes Association, as many as two out of three diabetic adults suffer from hypertension. Since type 2 diabetes can be effectively controlled through lifestyle changes, this is a problem that can be solved. This subject will be dealt with in detail in Chapter 7, which is dedicated to type 2 diabetes.

Medications

While they may be effective treatments for other conditions, certain traditional medications can actually cause hypertension. Although they are designed to reduce inflammation, corticosteroids, including prednisone and cortisone, and non-steroidal anti-inflammatory drugs (NSAIDs), including ibuprofen and aspirin, can actually increase blood pressure by constricting blood vessels. The same is true for migraine headache medications such as zolmitriptan (Zomig) and isometheptene (Midrin). Tricyclic antidepressants, including amitriptyline (Elavil) and protriptyline

(Vivactil), have also been known to cause hypertension over time. Common decongestants such as pseudoephedrine (Sudafed) and diphenhydramine (Benadryl) can raise blood pressure and reduce the effectiveness of blood pressure medication. Even hormone treatments, including estrogen replacement therapy and birth control pills, have been linked to an increase in blood pressure, as mentioned earlier. If you have been diagnosed with hypertension, it makes sense to discuss your medications with your doctor.

In addition to legal medications, illegal substances, including ecstasy, cocaine, and amphetamines, can also put you at risk for high blood pressure.

HOW DO YOU REDUCE THE RISK OF HYPERTENSION?

While the processes that result in hypertension may sound complicated, the simple truth is that high blood pressure occurs when levels of a select few chemical compounds are out of balance in the body. By keeping the amounts of these compounds in check, you can make significant strides towards a life without hypertension. Vitamin D_3 can play a powerful role in the regulation of blood pressure, as can omega-3 fatty acids. Most obviously, lifestyle choices, such as quitting smoking, getting exercise, and eating the right foods, can go a long way in combating this silent killer. Take advantage of the following information, so that you can reduce the risk of hypertension-related illness.

Take Vitamin D₃

As you now know, vitamin D_3 is responsible for keeping the body's production of the enzyme renin in check. A deficiency in this vitamin allows an overabundance of renin to wreak havoc in the renin-angiotensin-aldosterone system. The increase in renin stimulates production of angiotensin, which raises aldosterone levels, both of which result in high blood pressure. Taking an oral vitamin D_3 supplement can cure that deficiency, thus decreasing your chance of acquiring hypertension and the cardiovascular diseases associated with it. Since dark-skinned people require at least five times the amount of vitamin D_3 as light-skinned people, I recommend that African Americans take between 2,000 and 5,000 IU of the supplement. Always ask your doctor to check your vitamin D_3 levels, however, before starting supplementation.

Take Omega-3 Fatty Acids

To treat pain and inflammation, most people reach for traditional over-the-counter medications such as ibuprofen (Motrin), acetaminophen (Tylenol), or acetylsalicylic acid (Aspirin). Unfortunately, each of these choices can cause serious side effects over time, including bleeding, kidney damage, and even high blood pressure. Omega-3 fatty acids present an alternative method of treatment without the numerous downsides of traditional medications. Like vitamins, these fatty acids are required by the body but cannot be synthesized by it. They must therefore be acquired through diet or supplements.

Fish oil, flaxseed, and walnuts are a few of the dietary sources of omega-3 fatty acids. These fatty acids reduce inflammation, relieve pain, boost the effectiveness of other pain medications, and keep cell membranes from hardening. They also have a positive affect on nerve cells, protecting them against damage. Omega-3 fatty acids are usually sold in liquid or pill form. Dosage is dependent on your individual health condition, but I would generally recommend no less than 1,000 mg per day for adults and 250 to 500 mg per day for children. Research has shown that omega-3 fatty acid supplements can be taken in doses up to 2,000 mg per day without side effects in adults.

Change Your Diet

It should come as no surprise that a healthy diet can have a tremendously positive effect not only on your blood pressure but also on your overall well-being. Because diet is associated with a number of the other causes of hypertension, little changes here and there can produce significant results.

Stress, as you know, is quite literally a killer. It can easily lead to hypertension and cardiovascular disease. By cutting your intake of alcohol, caffeine, sugar, and salt, you reduce your body's adrenaline production and therefore its stress level. Similarly, by avoiding an abundance of high-protein animal foods, you decrease the anxiety-promoting compounds dopamine and nor-epinephrine in the brain. On the other end of the spectrum, foods that are high in complex carbohydrates and fiber can increase your levels of serotonin, the body's own calming chemical. The same can be said for eating more vegetables, which are rich in beneficial vitamins and minerals. Lowering your salt intake reduces hypertension caused by water retention, while decreasing your intake of fried and fatty foods will help cut your level of bad cholesterol, which in high amounts can result in plaque buildup along the walls of blood vessels, thereby raising blood pressure.

In fact, the above-mentioned food recommendations are officially promoted by the National Heart, Lung, and Blood Institute as the DASH (Dietary Approaches to Stop Hypertension) diet, which suggests eating fruit, vegetables, nuts, beans, and various lean meats while significantly limiting your intake of sugary beverages, fatty foods, and red meat.

Exercise

Exercise raises good cholesterol and lowers bad cholesterol, all the while helping you lose weight. The reduction in body mass benefits your blood pressure further by lightening the strain on your heart. Exercise also produces endorphins, which decrease stress levels. Finally, exercise lowers your blood sugar, thus helping you treat and even avoid another common cause of hypertension, type 2 diabetes. So, before you overwhelm yourself by considering all the medications you may one day have to take, simply go for a brisk thirty-minute walk five times a week. If you create a healthy fitness routine and stick to it, those medications may never be needed.

Quit Smoking

In addition to high blood pressure, smoking causes heart attacks, stroke, blood clots, numerous forms of cancer, and emphysema. So much has been written about this bad habit that I do not feel the need to say much more than this: Please quit smoking. If you lack the willpower to do so on your own, find some help. There are many new methods that can assist you in your goal. Cigarettes are a poison. Cut that poison out of your life.

Consider Other Supplements

Along with traditional medications and well-known vitamins, other supplements have proven helpful against hypertension. One of them is coenzyme Q_{10}, or CoQ_{10}, which aids in the body's creation of energy. A decline in this coenzyme has major affects on the heart, decreasing the amount of energy available for the heart to pump efficiently and continuously. Unfortunately, statin drugs, which are typically prescribed to combat high cholesterol, can interfere with the body's production and utilization of CoQ_{10}. To compensate for any loss of this coenzyme, you can take CoQ_{10} supplements of up to 100 mg, one to three times a day.

Another often overlooked supplement is hawthorn berry. Although knowledge of this berry goes back about 700 years, its medicinal use was only officially recognized in 1984, when the German Commission E showed that it could lower blood pressure by opening blood vessels. It is best used for people who do not yet have hypertension, though it can supplement already established treatment. The recommended daily dosage of hawthorn berry extract is 160 to 900 mg. As always, check with your doctor to be sure that the supplement does not interfere with any other medications you are taking.

CONCLUSION

Although you may not be able to eradicate your chances of acquiring hypertension completely, you can try your best to remedy and eliminate the factors that contribute to high blood pressure. While conventional drugs dominate traditional methods of treatment at the moment, they do not address the root causes of the condition. Abnormal functioning of the RAAS system, inflammation caused by elevated homocysteine levels, not to mention lifestyle factors such as stress, diet, and a lack of exercise, all form the basis of high blood pressure.

Thankfully, inexpensive supplements, including vitamin D_3 and omega-3 fatty acids, can be very effective in the alleviation of these underlying factors. In addition to supplements, regular exercise and a diet rich in vegetables, complex carbohydrates, and fiber will help you avoid a rise in blood pressure, while also improving your mood in general.

You must remember that hypertension does not just flare up once in while. It is a silent, ongoing condition, whose first symptom can be sudden death. As African Americans run a considerably higher risk than other segments of the population, I am strongly encouraging you to become more diligent in caring for yourself. You need to recognize all the factors that contribute to hypertension—especially those that particularly affect the black population, such as vitamin D_3 deficiency and stress. In doing so, you will be able to take full advantage of each and every method of treatment available.

5

Cancer

According to the US Department of Health and Human Services' Office of Minority Health, black Americans are far more likely to die of cancer than any other ethnic or racial group in the country. Compared to white males, African-American males are more likely to be diagnosed with lung, prostate, and stomach cancer, and have lower five-year survival rates in connection with lung and pancreatic cancer. Although African-American women are slightly less likely than their white counterparts to be diagnosed with breast cancer, they are much more likely to die of it. Their chance of acquiring stomach cancer is double that of white women, and they are twice as likely to die of the disease. These kinds of cancer rates cannot be ignored.

It would be nice if I could give a complete and simple explanation for these statistics, but unfortunately I cannot. When dealing with cancer, answers are often complex and hard to come by. But let us not discount the fact that there *are* some answers. One of those answers is the main subject of this book. There is convincing evidence that vitamin D_3 deficiency contributes to the formation and proliferation of cancer cells, which suggests that an increase in vitamin D_3 intake in the black community could potentially curb its staggering cancer rates. This information is vital to initiating a positive change in the health of African Americans, not to mention the country as a whole.

After first defining the nature of cancer and its known causes, this chapter will discuss the ways in which you can lower your risk. While focusing on vitamin D3 deficiency, it will also address a number of other cancer-related factors, many of which you can control. We must remember that statistics are subject to change. They are not the ultimate determinants of the future of black America. We *can* write our own story.

WHAT IS CANCER?

Cancer is the uncontrolled growth of abnormal cells in the body. It can arise from any type of cell in any organ. Whether caused by random error, inherited abnormality, or environmental factors called *carcinogens,* when the genetic information, or DNA, of a cell is damaged, that damage can produce mutations in the cell. If the mutated cell begins to reproduce itself without restriction, those abnormal cells often form a mass, or tumor, that may be cancerous.

Figure 5.1 on page 47 shows two types of cell division. The top example shows a mutated cell undergoing cellular suicide. Thankfully, one of the miracles of human life is that every single cell in the body is preprogrammed to self-destruct once it recognizes anything wrong with its development. It is a fortunate process called *apoptosis* and is initiated by the p53 gene, also known as the tumor-suppressing gene. If this gene is turned off because of damage or genetic abnormality, it will not allow the abnormal cell to recognize its mutation. The cell, therefore, will continue to survive and multiply.

The formation of a tumor, however, does not necessarily mean cancer. All tumors are not cancerous, though the words tumor and cancer are often used synonymously. When discussing tumors, the two most important terms to understand are malignant and benign. If a tumor is benign, it is not cancerous. This kind of tumor generally does not spread and, most of the time, does not return once removed. One example of a common benign tumor is uterine fibroids, which are small growths in the uterus. Malignant tumors, on the other hand, are cancerous. They have the potential

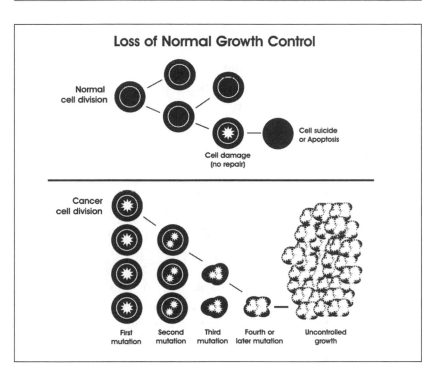

Figure 5.1. Normal versus Abnormal Cell Division.

to invade other tissues and spread throughout the body through a process called *metastasis*. While most cancers are marked by the presence of a tumor, some, such as leukemia, are not.

WHAT CAUSES CANCER?

The potential for cancer exists in your body as long as its cells are thriving and dividing, which is basically as long as you're alive. Imperfect cells that can cause cancer usually arise because of damage from free radicals. As previously mentioned in this book, these unstable molecules are some of the most destructive things that occur in your system. While they can be created by exposure to environmental factors called *carcinogens*, such as cigarette smoke and asbestos, they also spring up unavoidably through the natural functions of the body. Free radicals can sometimes injure the aforementioned p53 gene, turning it off and thereby allowing cancers to flourish.[1,2,3] In addition, inadequate levels of vitamin

D3 may result in cell abnormalities that have been associated with the first stage of cancer.

The onset of the disease has also been linked to genetic predisposition and even certain viruses. While some causes of cancer seem beyond our control, some can definitely be avoided. Below are a few of the major examples.

Vitamin D3 Deficiency

Recent research has linked the development of cancer to the loss of contact between cells, also known as *disjunction*. Essentially, when cells maintain proper contact with each other, their signals remain strong. This attachment helps them protect each other and may also increase the effectiveness of apoptosis. Vitamin D3 deficiency has proven to decrease the stickiness of cells, possibly leading to the growth of tumors and a reduction in the ability of these abnormal cells to self-destruct before becoming cancerous.

Even if your body produces sufficient amounts of vitamin D3 to prevent disjunction, frequent exposure to carcinogens such as tobacco smoke, industrial chemicals, and toxic mold, or simply a high intake of sugar in your diet can overwhelm the protective benefits of the nutrient.

Asbestos

Asbestos is a designation given to six fibrous minerals, each of which show a similar resistance to high heat and numerous chemicals. Because of these physical properties, asbestos was commonly used as insulation in schools, factories, and homes, before it was recognized as a cancer-causing substance. It was also used to make automobile parts, building materials, and even textiles. Shipbuilders during World War II as well as workers in factories that produced asbestos-containing products were particularly exposed to large amounts of asbestos dust, which remains in the lungs once breathed in. In addition to lung cancer, this dust can cause a type of cancer of the lung called *mesothelioma*. Although its use is not as widespread anymore, it may still be present in old homes and workplaces.

Cigarettes

While it is also associated with heart disease, lung disease, and stroke, cigarette smoke is most notably a cancer-causing agent. It contains hundreds of chemicals, dozens of which have been classified as carcinogens. These chemicals include arsenic, benzene, cadmium, nickel, ethylene oxide, and beryllium, to name just a few. Not only a leading cause of lung cancer, cigarette smoke has also been linked to many types of cancer in the body, including cancer of the kidneys and bladder.

Diet

There are a number of dietary factors that can influence your chance of getting cancer. A diet that is high in fat has consistently been associated with an increased risk of numerous forms of cancer, as well as with obesity, which is itself a cancer risk. Consuming alcohol raises your chance of acquiring a variety of cancers, including cancer of the mouth, liver, breast, and bowel. To a lesser degree, cancer has also been linked to high red meat intake, especially when the meat is cooked at a high temperature, such as on a barbeque, which releases certain chemicals that can damage your cells.

Genetic Predisposition

An inherited mutation of certain tumor-suppressing genes has been linked to the susceptibility of an individual to cancer. In addition, some scientists actually argue for the presence of a cancer-*causing* gene called an *oncogene,* which may be more likely to be activated in certain people than in others. But much more research must be done, and it is important to remember that having a predisposition to cancer is not a guarantee that you will one day acquire the disease.

Radiation

Radiation is essentially waves of energy that exist at different frequencies. High frequency radiation negatively affects your body by removing electrons from the atoms in your body, thereby creating free radicals, which can damage your DNA and ultimately result in cancer. This process is called *ionization*. Sources of ionizing radiation include cosmic rays, natural radiation from the earth, medical diagnostic tests, nuclear weapons, and, to a degree, ultraviolet light. While non-ionizing sources of radiation such as power lines, televisions, and cell phones have been called into question as possible carcinogens, no concrete link has yet been made between them and cancer.

Viruses

Though it is rare to acquire cancer from a virus, there are, nevertheless, a handful of viruses that have been linked to certain forms of the disease, such as the human t-cell lymphotrophic virus, which can lead to adult t-cell leukemia, and the human papillomavirus, which can lead to cervical cancer. The association between cervical cancer and the human papillomavirus is so strong, in fact, that the medical community suggests vaccination for girls as early as age nine, as the vaccine is most effective before a female has had any sexual contact.

HOW DO YOU REDUCE THE RISK OF CANCER?

Because vitamin D_3 has proven to have a protective effect on cells, a deficiency of this nutrient may prevent you from reducing your risk of cancer. Thankfully, you do not have to let vitamin D_3 deficiency stop you from being cancer-free. A little bit of sunshine and proper supplementation can easily raise your level of vitamin D_3. But simply dealing with this important nutrient is not enough. If you allow yourself to be exposed to too many environmental carcinogens, such as those mentioned above, these forces can eventually overwhelm even vitamin D_3's cancer-fighting properties.

Lifestyle choices, including quitting smoking and changing your diet, can certainly help you avoid the disease and retain the potency of vitamin D_3. In addition to the sunshine vitamin, adding a few other supplements, including vitamin K_2 and turmeric, can aid in the pursuit of living a life without cancer. With so many factors within our control, together we can significantly cut the cancer rates not only of the black community but also of the entire population of the country.

Take Vitamin D_3

What if I told you that there was a way to stop approximately 58,000 new cases of breast cancer, eliminate 49,000 new cases of colorectal cancer, and reduce the occurrence of prostate cancer by half every year? There is an abundance of scientific data which strongly suggest that increasing your vitamin D_3 level can achieve these results. Once considered only in terms of bone health, research now shows that all cells in the body have vitamin-D receptors that help control normal cell growth and attachment, and possibly even improve the effectiveness of apoptosis. But how much vitamin D_3 is enough?

The recommended amount of vitamin D_3, according to the Food and Drug Administration, is about 800 IU per day. From all the research I have read, however, this number is insufficient, even if you are light-skinned. Therefore, researchers and experts in the field recommend a minimum of 2,000 IU per day. Because the necessary amount naturally varies depending on the latitude at which you live (which, as you now know, affects your exposure to vitamin D-producing UVB rays) and the pigmentation of your skin (which affects UVB absorption), I generally recommend at least 5,000 IU per day for African Americans and other dark-skinned ethnic groups.

The best thing you can do is get your healthcare provider to order a blood test for vitamin D_3 levels. An optimal level of the nutrient falls between 50 and 80 ng/mL. You can simply adjust your supplements accordingly to reach those measurements.

There are over 3,000 studies showing the relationship between high levels of vitamin D_3 and lower rates of a variety of cancers. In what I believe was an unprecedented move, the researchers of one review article were so thoroughly convinced of the importance of vitamin D_3 that they included an open letter at the end of the published study, urging people to take adequate amounts of vitamin D_3. (See the inset on page 54.) There is certainly something big going on, and you need to hear about it. Let us look at the different types of cancer to see how vitamin D_3 can play a role in their prevention.

Breast Cancer

The results are clear. Reduced sunlight exposure is associated with lower levels of vitamin D_3 and higher incidences of breast cancer. Moreover, declines in breast cancer appear directly proportional to increased UVB sunlight exposure.[4] Studies have shown that women who maintain a vitamin D_3 level over 38 ng/mL also have a 58-percent lower risk of breast cancer than women whose vitamin D_3 level is below 15 ng/mL.[5]

According to a speech given by noted scientist Dr. Cedric Garland at a conference at the University of Toronto, a woman's risk of contracting breast cancer can be virtually eradicated by sufficiently elevating her vitamin D level. At this same conference, Dr. Garland presented data that displayed that an increase in vitamin D levels to near 80 ng/mL was associated with a decrease in breast cancer risk of more than 77 percent. Thirty of the world's leading researchers on vitamin D and many other vitamin D supporters recommend 2,000 IU of vitamin D daily, with a goal of reaching an average vitamin D blood level of 40 to 60 ng/mL.

Prostate Cancer

It is estimated that at least half of US men age sixty and over have prostate cancer. According to the American Cancer Society, prostate cancer is the second most prevalent cancer in men after lung cancer, and represents at least 10 percent of male cancer-related deaths.[6] Because the disease often has no symptoms, it can go unnoticed for years, sometimes remaining undetected for life, provided it is of the non-aggressive variety. An aggressive form of the disease is very hard to treat, as it has usually spread to other organs by the time of its diagnosis.[7]

As with breast cancer, research has shown that low levels of vitamin D_3 are directly related to high rates of prostate cancer. Even more importantly, vitamin D deficiency has been associated with an increase in the occurrence of the aggressive form of the disease. This troubling statistic is of particular concern for dark-skinned men, who frequently suffer from low levels of the nutrient. During the winter months, rates of less than 24 ng/mL of vitamin D_3 in men are considered low. During the summer months, amounts of less than 32 ng/mL of vitamin D_3 in men also suggest a deficiency.[8]

Colorectal Cancer

Colorectal cancer occurs in the large intestine, specifically the colon and rectum. The appearance of small growths called *polyps* along the surface of the colon and rectum is an early warning sign of the disease. The presence of these polyps is what doctors look for during a colonoscopy exam. If they are found and determined to be malignant, treatment is necessary. It is recommended that everyone get regular colonoscopy exams after age fifty, especially those people who have a family history of the illness.

According to research, the relationship between vitamin D_3 concentrations and reductions in colorectal cancer diagnoses and deaths is dramatic. Patients with vitamin D_3 blood levels greater than 32 ng/mL have a 75-percent chance of fully recovering from the disease, [9,10,11] while those who have rates above 38 ng/mL reduce their chance of contracting colorectal cancer by 55 percent.[12]

Ovarian and Endometrial Cancer

The effect of vitamin D_3 on ovarian and endometrial cancer is very impressive. As you might suspect, when exposure to UVB light increases, levels of vitamin D_3 also increase, while the rates of both of these cancers of the female reproductive system drop.[13,14,15] What is of particular note when discussing vitamin D's effect on endometrial cancer, which occurs in the lining of the uterus, is its effectiveness in the presence of cancer-promoting factors such as excess weight, diabetes, poor diet, and family history. Even with

Scientists' Letter on Vitamin D for Cancer and other Disease Prevention

The following is an open letter provided by the researchers of the review article "Vitamin D for Cancer Prevention: Global Perspective."[16] They included this plea in their study in an effort to illuminate the importance of vitamin D_3 to the greater medical establishment and declare it an urgent matter.

To Whom It May Concern:

We are aware of substantial scientific evidence supporting the role of vitamin D in prevention of cancer. It has been reasonably established that adequate serum vitamin D metabolite levels are associated with substantially lower incidence rates of several types of cancer, including those of the breast, colon, and ovary, and other sites.

We have concluded that the vitamin D status of most individuals in North America will need to be greatly improved for substantial reduction in incidence of cancer. Epidemiological studies have shown that higher vitamin D levels are also associated with lower risk of Type I diabetes in children and of multiple sclerosis. Several studies have found that markers of higher vitamin D levels are associated with lower incidence and severity of influenza and several other infectious diseases.

Higher vitamin D status can be achieved in part by increased oral intake of vitamin D_3. The appropriate intake of vitamin D_3 for cancer risk reduction depends on the individual's age, race, lifestyle, and latitude of residence. New evidence indicates that the intake should be 2000 IU per day. Intake of 2000 IU/day is the current upper limit of the National Academy of Sciences, Institute of Medicine, Food and Nutrition Board. New evidence also indicates that the upper limit should be raised substantially. The levels that are needed to prevent a substantial proportion of cancer would also be effective in substantially reducing risk of fractures, Type I childhood diabetes and multiple sclerosis.

Greater oral intakes of vitamin D_3 may be needed in the aged and in individuals who spend little time outdoors, because of reduced cutaneous synthesis. Choice of a larger dose may be based on the individual's wintertime serum 25(OH)D level.

For those choosing to have serum 25-hydroxyvitamin D tested, a target serum level should be chosen in consultation with a health care provider, based on the characteristics of the individual. An approximate guide-line for health care providers who choose to measure serum 25-hydroxyvitamin D in their patients would to aim for 40–60 ng/ml, unless there are specific contraindications. Contraindications are extremely rare, and are well known to physicians. No intervention is free of all risk, including this one. Patients should be advised of this, and advised in detail of risks that may be specific to the individual.

Any risks of vitamin D inadequacy considerably exceed any risks of taking 2000 IU/day of vitamin D_3, which the NAS-IOM regards as having no adverse health effect.

A substantially higher level of support for research on the role of vitamin D for the prevention of cancer is urgently needed. However, delays in taking reasonable preventive action on cancer by ensuring nearly universal oral intake of vitamin D_3 of 2000 IU/day is costing thousands of lives unnecessarily each year that are lost due to fractures, cancer, diabetes, multiple sclerosis, and other diseases for which vitamin D deficiency plays a major role.

Signed:

Cedric F. Garland, Dr.P.H., F.A.C.E., Professor (Adj), UC San Diego

Frank C. Garland, Ph.D., Professor (Adj), UC San Diego

Edward Giovannucci, M.D., Sc.D, Professor, Harvard School of Public Health

Edward D. Gorham, M.P.H., Ph.D., Assistant Professor, UC San Diego

William B. Grant, Ph.D., Sunlight, Nutrition, and Health Research Center (SUNARC)

John Hathcock, Vice President Scientific and International Affairs, Council for Responsible Nutrition

Robert P. Heaney, M.D., Professor, Creighton University

Michael F. Holick, Ph.D., M.D., Director, Vitamin D, Skin and Bone Research Laboratory, Boston University School of Medicine

Bruce W. Hollis, Ph.D., Director of Pediatric Nutritional Sciences, Medical University of South Carolina

Joan M. Lappe, Ph.D., R.N., F.A.A.N., Professor, Creighton University

Anthony W. Norman, Ph.D., Distinguished Professor, UC Riverside

Reinhold Vieth Ph.D., F.C.A.C.B., Professor, University of Toronto all of these cancer-contributors taken into consideration, vitamin D_3 still lowers your risk of this illness.[17]

Take Vitamin K_2

While researching bone loss in women with cirrhosis of the liver, Japanese scientists stumbled across data that suggested vitamin K_2 as a measure of prevention against liver cancer. To their surprise, women who had been given a vitamin K_2 supplement were 90 percent less likely to develop liver cancer, a common result of cirrhosis of the liver, than those who had not.

A German study also proved a link between increased levels of vitamin K_2 and a decrease in prostate cancer in men. The recommended daily allowance of this vitamin is 70 to 80 mcg per day for men, and 55 to 65 mcg per day for women.

Take Omega-3 Fatty Acids

Omega-3 fatty acids are necessary to maintain good health but cannot be manufactured by the body. They must be obtained through diet—usually by eating fish—or supplementation. Some studies have shown that adults who maintain an omega-3 fatty acid intake of 1 to 3 grams per day are less likely to develop cancer of the colon, breast, and prostate.

Take Green Tea Extract

Made from unfermented tea leaves, green tea contains antioxidants called *polyphenols*. The majority of the polyphenols found in green tea fall into a group of compounds called *catechins*, which seem to prevent cancer cells from growing and spreading. I recommend adding 6 to 9 drops of green tea extract to 32 ounces of water and drinking the mixture throughout the day.

Take Turmeric (Curcumin)

Turmeric is a spice commonly used in Indian cuisine. Its most biologically active component, curcumin, has become known for its potential anti-cancer behavior. One of the most amazing things about curcumin is that it seems to stop the progression of cancer cells while ignoring healthy cells. While more research is required to determine the optimal amount of supplementation, 250 mg twice daily is considered an appropriate dosage of curcumin extract, although people have been known to take higher doses. The most typical side effects of high dosages include nausea and diarrhea. Curcumin should not be taken by individuals undergoing chemotherapy, as it may make the treatment less effective.

Take Probiotics

Also referred to as "friendly bacteria," probiotics are microorganisms that live in the digestive tract and regulate the growth of harmful bacteria. By inhibiting the proliferation of potentially cancer-promoting bacteria, neutralizing other carcinogenic agents, and boosting the immune system, probiotics are thought to be especially protective against colon cancer. Common daily dosages of probiotics range from 2 to 10 billion live bacteria, acquired from dietary supplements or by eating foods such as yogurt. If you are undergoing chemotherapy, talk to your doctor before taking probiotic supplements.

Quit Smoking

As I mentioned in the last chapter, smoking is one of the unhealthiest things you could do to your body. The link between cigarettes and numerous types of cancer has been solidly established. It seems like every year, this nasty habit is connected to yet another form of the disease. Quitting smoking is probably the single best thing you could do to lower your cancer risk. If you are a smoker, please do not wait another day to stop.

Change Your Diet

Research suggests that lowering the amount of fat in your diet also lowers your risk of contracting colon, prostate, and breast cancer. Studies also show an association between diets that are high in fiber and decreased rates of stomach and colorectal cancer. In addition, populations that consume lots of fruits, vegetables, and whole grains consistently display lower rates of numerous forms of cancer than those that do not. Finally, there is evidence that the higher a population's intake of animal protein, the higher its rates of numerous cancers are. Perhaps the most compelling source of this research can be found in Dr. T. Colin Campbell's book *The China Study: Startling Implications for Diet, Weight Loss and Long-Term Health,* which argues that a vegan diet can help you avoid cancer.

CONCLUSION

I hope that this chapter has given you a sense of optimism in the face of the African-American community's high rates of cancer. Although the statistics are bleak, there is truly no reason that you cannot change them for the better. By increasing your vitamin D_3 level, you can ensure that your body is able to destroy potentially cancerous cells before they multiply. Add to that some of the exciting new research on other cancer-fighting supplements, and you can begin to turn the tide on some of the most common cancers affecting black Americans, including colon, prostate, and lung cancer. In addition, by adopting healthy lifestyle habits and trying your best to avoid environmental carcinogens, you can make great strides towards a cancer-free lifetime, while ensuring that the protective mechanisms of vitamin D_3 and any other supplements remain effective. Although this information is absolutely vital for dark-skinned people to recognize, it is also of great benefit to all people, and applies to a wide variety of cancers.

6

Stroke

troke is the third greatest cause of death and the leading cause of adult disability in the United States. The occurrence of stroke doubles every decade after the age of 55. According to a University of Michigan study, the cost of caring for victims of stroke in this country will amount to $2.2 trillion over the next 45 years, unless we all do more to lower our risk of stroke and improve stroke recovery. The majority of this cost will land on the shoulders of African-American and Latino stroke victims, who suffer twice as many strokes as their white counterparts, tend to have them at much younger ages, and get poorer quality preventive care than others. As stated by the study, half of the predicted total of stroke-related costs, which include ambulances, hospitalizations, medications, nursing home care, at-home care, visits to the doctor, and lost income, will come from people under the age of sixty-five.[1]

But this statistic is simply too big to grasp on an individual level. It does not explain the emotional cost to the victim and his loved ones—the stress, worry, pressure, and damage to the quality of life suffered by everyone involved. The total cost cannot truly be assessed. It can, however, be alleviated. The following chapter will tell you what exactly a stroke is, the causes behind stroke, and the steps you can take to avoid being the victim of a stroke—most of which are relatively simple modifications to your lifestyle.

WHAT IS A STROKE?

Much like a heart attack results from a disturbance in the blood flow in the heart, a stroke is the result of interrupted blood flow to the brain, which is why it is sometimes referred to as a "brain attack." This interruption, technically known as a *cerebrovascular accident*, causes a loss of brain function, which often results in paralysis of one side of the body, difficulty with language and speech, problems with vision, and memory loss. (See Figure 6.1.) While recovery is sometimes possible with the help of rehabilitation and therapy, it rarely ends with the victim regaining full function. There are two major types of stroke, each characterized by the way in which the attack manifests itself.

A Stroke's Effects on the Brain

The amount of neurological deficits caused by a stroke is directly determined by the location affected and the extent of the damage. The illustration below shows which areas of the brain control specific functions of the body.

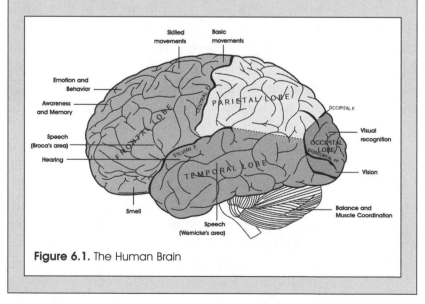

Figure 6.1. The Human Brain

Ischemic strokes are the most common type, accounting for about 85 percent of all cases. They are defined by a blood clot in a vessel that supplies blood to the brain. While the clot typically begins in the brain, it can also develop in any part of the circulatory system that has accumulated fatty deposits. In this case, a piece of the clot breaks off and makes its way to the brain until it reaches a blood vessel that is too small to allow for its passage, thus causing a stroke.

Hemorrhagic strokes make up about 15 percent of all cases. They are characterized by bleeding rather than clotting. The bleeding occurs either in the brain itself or between the brain and the skull, and is caused by a weakened blood vessel that has finally burst. The accumulation of blood puts pressure on the brain, while the discontinuation of blood to other areas of the brain depletes those regions of oxygen. Both types of stroke lead to the same loss of function.

In addition to the major kinds of stroke, it is very important to recognize a warning stroke, or "mini stroke." Medically dubbed a *transient ischemic attack,* or TIA, this minor attack has all the symptoms of a regular stroke, but lasts only a few minutes, as the blockage is only temporary. Unlike major strokes, TIA does not permanently damage the brain. It is, however, a wake-up call, as those who suffer a TIA usually fall victim to a full-blown stroke within one year.

WHAT CAUSES A STROKE?

According to the National Stroke Association, 80 percent of strokes are completely avoidable through lifestyle changes alone. Studies have shown that hypertension and diabetes increase the probability of stroke four fold, while smoking doubles it. Other contributors include atherosclerosis, elevated homocysteine levels, inactivity, obesity, and hormone replacement.[2] Many of these factors, in fact, are interrelated, which means that eliminating one of them would also help eliminate the others. For example, bringing your diabetes under control would also help reduce your risk of high blood pressure, which would help decrease your risk of atherosclerosis and atherosclerosis-related stroke. By addressing the root causes of stroke, you can help to lower your risk of this illness drastically.

Atherosclerosis

Atherosclerosis is a hardening of the arteries due to a buildup of plaque inside these blood vessels. When blood vessels accumulate too much cholesterol, that cholesterol hardens into plaque. Once the plaque becomes so thick that it narrows the walls of the affected blood vessel, blood clots are more likely to get stuck in that vessel, stopping blood flow and thus causing a stroke. (See Figure 6.2.) Since the blood vessels of the brain have the ability to alter their diameter as well as adjust blood flow to bypass obstructed areas, a stroke is not a guarantee for atherosclerosis patients. But make no mistake. The condition is linked to approximately half of all occurrences of stroke. Research has shown that the risk of atherosclerosis-related stroke is associated not only with elevated LDL cholesterol in the body but also with high levels of non-fast-

Figure 6.2. Atherosclerosis: Blood Vessel Cross-Sections.

Note the decreased size of the opening for blood flow in the artery shown on the right. The thickening along the vessel walls is atherosclerosis.

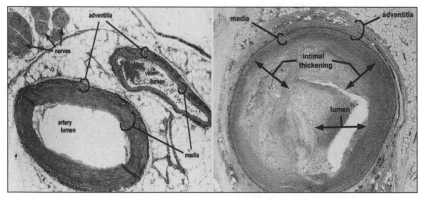

A. Cross section of normal artery and vein.

B. Cross section of artery with atherosclerosis.

From: Southern Ill. Univ. School of Med. www.siumed.edu

ing triglycerides, which indicate the presence of a type of cholesterol called *remnant lipoprotein.*

While cholesterol is a factor in atherosclerosis, it is not, however, the root cause. (See the inset below.) As you will soon see, atherosclerosis is closely associated with a number of other risk factors for stroke, a great number of which lead to an attack by first causing a buildup of plaque in your arteries.

The True Cause of Atherosclerosis

While high cholesterol often takes the rap for atherosclerosis, it is important to recall that cholesterol is the building block of a number of crucial chemical compounds in the body, including hormones such as estrogen, progesterone, and testosterone, not to mention the subject of this book, vitamin D_3. Thanks to television ads, however, you probably know cholesterol only in relation to the idea of plaque buildup. Although it is true that cholesterol is closely linked to atherosclerosis, it is not the source of the problem. If you were to completely correct high cholesterol with typically prescribed drugs, called *statins,* you'd remedy only about 25 percent of all cases. This is because statin drugs do not treat the chief culprit behind the condition: inflammation.

Inflammation, not cholesterol, is the root cause of the majority of cases of atherosclerosis.[3,4,5,6] Inflammation in the body can be caused by such things as free radicals, elevated levels of an amino acid called *homocysteine,* chronic infections,[7,8] heavy metal toxicity,[9,10,11,12] and even allergies.[13] Inflammation damages a layer of cells called the *endolethium,* which lines the interior walls of blood vessels. These damaged cells attract white blood cells, which attempt to stop the inflammation. Unfortunately, they are often unable to do so and ultimately rupture, creating more damage and inflammation. Thus begins a cascade of other rapidly destructive effects. The immune system begins to secrete proteins called *cytokines,* which regulate the body's response to biological invaders, allergens, and trauma. These cytokines promote even further inflammation of the endolethium. It is at this point where cholesterol comes into play. Cholesterol begins to accumulate in the area of damage. Over time, it causes the interior lining of the affected blood vessel to harden, narrowing the area through which blood can flow.

Hypertension

People with hypertension, also known as high blood pressure, are four to six times more likely to have a stroke. This is a staggering statistic for African Americans, one third of whom suffer from the condition. High blood pressure is especially dangerous because it often occurs without symptoms, damaging your body silently until it is too late.

Hypertension leads to stroke by contributing to and accelerating the buildup of plaque in the arteries due to atherosclerosis. It can also cause a piece of plaque to break off and become lodged in a blood vessel in the brain, resulting in an ischemic stroke, or weaken a blood vessel so much that it bursts, resulting in a hemorrhagic stroke.

Diabetes

The risk of stroke is two to four times higher for people with diabetes than those without the disease. Diabetics are also three times more likely to die of stroke than non-diabetics. The elevated glucose levels associated with diabetes significantly contribute to the buildup of plaque in your body. Most diabetics also suffer from hypertension, which, as previously explained, worsens the risk of stroke that accompanies atherosclerosis. Latinos and African Americans are approximately twice as likely as white people to be diagnosed with diabetes.

Elevated Homocysteine Levels

Elevated levels of an amino acid called homocysteine are known to cause inflammation of the blood vessels. Unfortunately, this reaction produces a powerful domino effect that eventually leads to clogged arteries and high blood pressure, each of which substantially increases your risk of stroke. High levels of this amino acid have been linked to a deficiency in vitamins B_6, B_9, and B_{12}. Such a deficiency can be caused by a diet that lacks foods such as leafy greens, fortified grain products, and beans, all of which are good sources of B vitamins. It can also be a symptom of kidney disease and low thyroid function, not to mention the use of certain medications that can block your body's absorption of B vitamins. These medications include cholesterol-reducing drugs, antibiotics, non-steroidal anti-inflammatory drugs, and even caffeine.

Smoking

A smoker's risk of stroke is more than double that of a non-smoker. In addition to damaging the walls of your blood vessels, the chemicals found in cigarettes, including nicotine and carbon monoxide, lower the amount of oxygen in your blood. The habit increases your blood pressure and your chance of acquiring blood clots, thus raising the likelihood that you will suffer a stroke.

Obesity

Studies show that your risk of stroke increases as your level of obesity increases. This relationship may be a result of obesity being a significant contributor to hypertension and diabetes, both of which can lead to stroke.[14]

Birth Control and Hormone Replacement

One of the possible side effects of taking birth control pills is blood clots. Women who are smokers, over thirty-five years old, overweight, diabetic, or have high blood pressure run the highest risk of this side effect, although it has happened to a number of women who did not fit this profile. Even when using a low-dose birth control pill, the chance of stroke still exists.

There is also a slightly increased risk of stroke in women who undergo hormone replacement therapy. Most often used by women to treat symptoms of menopause, hormone treatments contain estrogen, which can create unwanted blood clots in much the same way that the estrogen in birth control pills can. Hormone replacement therapy is also associated with a modest elevation in the incidence of breast cancer in women. To take advantage of the benefits of hormones while avoiding their risks, always talk to your doctor before starting a hormone regimen of any kind.

HOW DO YOU REDUCE THE RISK OF A STROKE?

Although stroke is one of the leading killers in the United States, it is also one of the most preventable conditions that we face. A majority of its contributing factors, including hypertension, atherosclerosis, type 2 diabetes, and obesity, are controllable through lifestyle choices alone. By supplementing your diet with a few vitamins, maintaining a healthy weight, getting some exercise, and quitting smoking, you can virtually erase the threat of stroke from your life. The following simple modifications to your daily routine are things that everyone can and should do—especially African Americans, who account for such a large percentage of stroke victims in this country.

Exercise

Researchers have found that exercise reduces the occurrence not only of heart disease but also of stroke. Exercise raises your good cholesterol, lowers your blood pressure, and helps you lose weight, all of which are associated with decreasing your likelihood of stroke. Data suggests that people who engage in moderate exercise actually cut their risk of ischemic stroke in half. All it takes is a brisk thirty-minute walk five times a week to achieve positive results. Studies have also shown that stroke victims who had been physically active prior to their attack reported much milder symptoms than those who had not, while they also showed noticeably better rates of recovery.

Lose Weight

Being overweight is associated with so many of the contributing factors of stroke, including high blood pressure, high cholesterol, and diabetes. Research suggests that a reduction of weight by 5 to 10 percent can decrease your risk of stroke considerably. Thankfully, if you engage in exercise to lose weight, you will not only receive the protective benefits of the weight loss, but also of the physical activity itself.

Take Vitamin D₃

According to a recent study, there is a direct relationship between low levels of vitamin D_3 and the occurrence of stroke. In fact, the study goes so far as to declare vitamin D_3 deficiency an independent predictor of stroke. In other words, even when all other factors are excluded, insufficient amounts of vitamin D_3 are associated with an elevated number of strokes.[15,16] Although more research is required to determine the nature of this link, we do know that low vitamin D_3 levels promote hypertension and atherosclerosis, two of the most common contributors to stroke.

The study also suggests that vitamin D_3 supplementation may help you avoid a stroke. I recommend adding a vitamin D_3 supplement to your diet in the amount of 2,000 IU for light-skinned individuals and 5,000 IU for dark-skinned individuals.

Take B Vitamins

As discussed earlier, moderately high levels of an amino acid called homocysteine are associated with an elevated risk of stroke.[17] Due to their ability to lower homocysteine levels, B vitamins can be a useful tool against stroke. Although the effectiveness of B vitamins in decreasing the general incidence of stroke is still up for debate, studies have shown that they may reduce the chance of stroke in high-risk individuals, as well as stroke-related death.

In 1998, the United States and Canada began fortifying grain products with folic acid, also known as vitamin B_9.[18] Death rates due to stroke were studied before and after the fortification, and subsequently compared to England and Wales, where folic acid had not been added to the food supply. Results showed an increase in folate levels and a decrease in homocysteine levels in those populations whose food was fortified. They also showed a reduction of stroke-related deaths by approximately 13,000 per year in the United States, with a similar decline observed in Canada. The stroke statistics showed no decrease in England or Wales,[19] leading researchers to conclude that folic acid has a protective effect against stroke.

Since that time, it has also been suggested that a combination of B_6, B_9, and B_{12} may be even more effective. In addition, Vitamin B_3 (also known as niacin) may help lower bad cholesterol, which often sticks to the walls of blood vessels that have already been damaged by inflammation. Talk to your doctor about vitamin B supplementation, especially if your risk of stroke is high. Even without increased risk, I suggest getting at least the recommended daily intake of these nutrients, which amounts to about 15 mg of B_3, 2 mg of B_6, 400 mcg of B_9, and 2.4 mcg of B_{12}.

Quit Smoking

Smoking is one of the major contributors to your risk of stroke. Thankfully, smoking is also a habit that can be controlled and broken. Studies have shown that your chance of having a stroke decreases significantly and consistently immediately after you quit. Former smokers display the same risk of stroke as those who have never smoked after only five to fifteen years of being smoke-free.

CONCLUSION

Of all the diseases that are ravaging black America, stroke has some of the most interrelated causes. As a result, the ways in which you can reduce your risk of stroke are also interrelated, and should be approached together in order to achieve the most effective results. By combining vitamin supplements—specifically vitamin D_3 as well as vitamins B_3, B_6, B_9, and B_{12}—with regular exercise, a healthy weight, and a smoke-free lifestyle, you can alleviate and even avoid the most common contributors to stroke, including atherosclerosis, hypertension, obesity, and type 2 diabetes. And although it may depress you to realize that all of the recently mentioned illnesses have become signature conditions of the black community, it should encourage you to know that they are also within your control to avoid. You do not have to become another unfortunate statistic.

7

Type 2 Diabetes

What if you knew that on a certain day and time someone was going to rob your house and injure your family members? What if you also knew which of your things the thief would steal and which specific injuries would be suffered by your family? Would you take any and all preventative action in your power to protect them? I am certain you would. Type 2 diabetes should be looked upon in the exact same way. The warning signs of the disease are known, the kind of damage it inflicts upon your body is predictable, and preventive measures can be taken to stop it. Type 2 diabetes steals your organs, your limbs, your quality of life, your finances, and finally your life itself. The question is: What are you doing to stop it?

Type 2 diabetes is an expensive chronic disease. Diabetics use hospital emergency rooms twice as often as those without the disease.[1] This disorder is the major cause of adult blindness, non-traumatic lower-extremity amputations, and end-stage renal disease.[2] In addition, it has been observed that 80 percent of all deaths due to diabetes are actually the result of the cardiovascular diseases caused by the illness.[3] According to the American Diabetes Association, approximately 23.6 million Americans, or almost 8 percent of the population, have diabetes. Approximately 57 million Americans have prediabetes, which is defined by a number of conditions that precede the onset of full-blown type 2 diabetes.

While type 2 diabetes is generally considered an adult-onset illness, it is becoming more and more common in young people— a fact that coincides with the rising prevalence of childhood obesity. Although the disease continues to occur predominantly in those over forty years old, the fastest growing group being diagnosed is adolescents.[4] And despite the fact that we are living longer than ever before, the frequency of diabetes overall is growing right along with us.

The rate of type 2 diabetes in the black population of the United States is approximately double that of the white population. This fact is consistent not only with the number of diagnoses but also with the degree of severity of the illness, not to mention the amount of resultant deaths. Thankfully, many of the causative factors for type 2 diabetes can be reversed or avoided, no matter the color of your skin.

WHAT IS DIABETES?

Diabetes, also known as diabetes mellitus, is a condition defined by the body's inability to take glucose—its primary source of fuel—from the blood for use in the creation of energy. It is most clearly marked by an elevation in blood sugar. The illness is characterized by either a lack of the glucose-regulating hormone *insulin* or a decrease in the body's ability to use insulin properly. There are three types of diabetes—type 1 diabetes, type 2 diabetes, and gestational diabetes—though the main concern of this chapter will be type 2.

Type 1 Diabetes

Produced by the pancreas, insulin is a hormone required for the metabolism of glucose, also known as sugar. The effective use of glucose is essential for the body's survival. Simply put, none of the cells of the body can function without this energy source. In type 1 diabetes, the pancreas does not make insulin, which forces the victim to regulate his blood sugar through daily injections of the hormone. Type 1 diabetes is a genetically acquired disease considered by some doctors to be triggered by environmental causes. What those environmental causes may be is still an uncertainty, though research has found a possible connection between low levels of vitamin D and the onset of the illness, suggesting that a deficiency in the nutrient may allow the diabetes-causing genes to "turn on."[5] Although this type is not the focus of this chapter, the aforementioned link is worth noting.

Type 2 Diabetes

Type 2 diabetes accounts for almost 95 percent of all cases of diabetes in the United States. Unlike type 1, which occurs when the pancreas fails to produce insulin, type 2 sufferers have available insulin in their bodies, but their cell membranes have become unresponsive to it, resulting in a condition called *hyperinsulinemia,* or insulin resistance. Although there is definitely a genetic factor at play in type 2, the main risk factors for the illness are environmental triggers, including poor diet, inactivity, excessive weight, and low levels of vitamin D_3. Because the disease most often appears later in life, it has been called "adult-onset diabetes." Sadly, the increasing number of children and adolescents acquiring type 2 diabetes are causing that nickname to become less and less valid.

Gestational Diabetes

When a previously non-diabetic woman begins to show high blood sugar levels during pregnancy, she will be diagnosed with gestational diabetes. Scientists suspect that the hormones produced during pregnancy may increase a woman's resistance to insulin. While the new mother's system returns to normal once she has given birth, gestational diabetes may be an indicator of future type 2 diabetes.

The Destructive Nature of Diabetes

Both type 1 and type 2 diabetes have the same long-term destructive potential. Even when they are controlled through the use of medication, both conditions slowly wreak havoc on your system over time. Diabetes actually begins to damage your body—primarily your heart, brain, and kidneys—years before a diagnosis is made.[6,7] That damage is mainly the result of a process called *glycation*, which eventually causes a hardening of the arteries known as atherosclerosis, and atherosclerosis-related cardiovascular disease.

Glycation happens when sugar molecules bind to proteins or fats in the body, creating harmful compounds called *advanced glycation end products*, or AGEs. AGEs occur naturally in everyone, but their number and rate of production are accelerated by the excess glucose of a diabetic. A diagnosis of diabetes is, in fact, determined by the amount of hemoglobin molecules that have attached to sugar molecules (resulting in an AGE called HbA1c) over a three to six month period. AGEs impair cellular function and create free radicals, which in turn create oxidative stress and inflammation in your body.

It is with inflammation that we connect diabetes to cardiovascular illnesses, which can so easily take your life. Inflammation leads to atherosclerosis, and atherosclerosis can lead to strokes and heart attacks, as we have learned in previous chapters. Unfortunately, diabetes often goes hand in hand with hypertension, which increases your risk of cardiovascular disease even further. This fact is especially problematic for the black population, which has extremely high rates of high blood pressure already.

Because its origins are still not fully understood, type 1 diabetes remains seemingly unavoidable. Although there may be some encouraging evidence that suggests a preventative role for vitamin D_3, much more research is required. On the other hand, type 2 diabetes is essentially a disease of lifestyle that can be treated and perhaps even eradicated through adjustments to your daily routine.

As I asked at the beginning of this chapter, if you knew that a thief was on his way to rob you, and you knew exactly the way in which he was going to do so, not to mention what he was planning on taking from you, wouldn't you do everything you could to stop him from even showing up in the first place? Diabetes is a thief that gives you warnings, and if you take heed of them early, you can prevent its arrival altogether. By learning how to predict the illness, you can save yourself a lifetime of trouble.

WHAT CAUSES TYPE 2 DIABETES?

Perhaps no other disease has such obvious causative factors that can be addressed through changes in lifestyle, or such distinct warning signs that let you know there is still time to make those important changes. A family history of diabetes, your weight, and your level of physical activity are all things to consider. Even low levels of vitamin D_3 may play a role in the illness. And when these things are ignored, your body will set off alarm bells in the form of a number of conditions that, when occurring in combination, are called the *metabolic syndrome.* This syndrome includes high blood pressure, elevated blood glucose levels, and low HDL, or "good," cholesterol.

Family History

If a member of your family has type 2 diabetes, it is likely that you have a genetic predisposition to the disease. While a family history of the disease is one of the biggest risks for acquiring it, the predisposition seems only to affect those living a certain way. Unfortunately, that way is the typical Western lifestyle of overeating and getting little physical activity. This fact is especially important for African Americans families, so many of which have a long history of diabetes.

Obesity

There is an overwhelming link between being overweight and falling victim to type 2 diabetes. Studies suggest that the accumulation of body fat—particularly around the midsection—causes insulin resistance in cells, resulting in a rise in blood sugar levels. Research also shows that glucose metabolism improves significantly with the loss of excess weight. Unfortunately, most of the foods that promote easy weight gain—processed food, soda, refined flour and sugar—have become staples of the American diet. This type of diet harms not only adults, but children as well, more and more of whom are succumbing to obesity-related diabetes every day.

Sedentary Lifestyle

Acting hand in hand with the obesity epidemic in this country, a sedentary lifestyle contributes to the formation of type 2 diabetes. Studies show a decrease in insulin sensitivity in inactive people—a group which, sadly, includes most Americans. While most of the population engages in very little physical activity on a daily basis, almost a quarter of Americans get no exercise at all. Like obesity, this problem is starting to affect children as well as adults.

Sleep Habits

According to the first National Health and Nutrition Examination Survey, people who get less than five hours of sleep per night are at an increased risk for type 2 diabetes. Similar to the effects of inactivity and obesity, a failure to get the recommended seven to eight hours of sleep per night can result in insulin resistance, increasing the demand on the pancreas and raising blood sugar.

Vitamin D$_3$ Deficiency

Every day, more and more evidence connects low levels of vitamin D$_3$ with diabetes and diminished control of the disease. Defects found in vitamin D receptor (VDR) genes have proven to result in two types of genetic variants, also called *polymorphisms*. Characterized by weaker substitutes of original genes, polymorphisms create difficulties in the cellular functions of your body. One of these genetic variants is linked to excessive weight gain, while the other is linked to impaired insulin sensitivity and low levels of "good" cholesterol (HDL).[8] In addition, vitamin D$_3$ deficiency may also cause an increase in parathyroid hormone, which promotes insulin resistance and is associated with diabetes, hypertension, inflammation, and thus cardiovascular disease.[9] Research also suggests that obese children and adolescents have a higher risk of developing abnormal blood sugar when their vitamin D_3 levels are low.[10] Finally, statistics show that African Americans and Latinos display poorer control of the disease than whites, which I suspect has much to do with the increased effort it takes for dark skin to synthesize sunlight into vitamin D_3.

Metabolic Syndrome

As many people are still unfamiliar with the issue, no discussion about diabetes should go without mentioning the *metabolic syndrome,* previously known as syndrome X. As opposed to the disease itself, this syndrome is a group of symptoms that precedes the onset of type 2 diabetes. The presence of three or more of the following five symptoms is required for a diagnosis of metabolic syndrome to be made. They include high triglyceride levels, low HDL cholesterol levels, high blood pressure, high blood glucose levels, and a waist circumference of more than 40 inches for a man or 35 inches for a woman.

Although technically not a part of the metabolic syndrome, another predictor of diabetes is a darkening of the skin around the neck or armpits known as *acanthosis nigricans.* The discoloration of the skin indicates high levels of insulin in the blood, which suggests insulin resistance in the body. Sadly, many of these criteria are now being found in children.

HOW DO YOU REDUCE THE RISK OF DIABETES?

Reducing your risk of type 2 diabetes has one accepted simple formula: Shed excess weight, engage in regular physical activity, and get some sleep. Couple these lifestyle modifications with an increased intake of vitamin D_3 as well as a few other supplements and you are well on your way to stopping the destructive thief that is type 2 diabetes from entering your body and stealing your good health.

Exercise

Every time you exercise, your body requires extra energy, which it takes in the form of glucose in your blood. Any brief period of physical activity will do it, but continuous moderate exercise raises your body's use of glucose by twenty times its normal rate. This is how physical effort lowers your blood sugar.

Studies show that strength training, such as weight lifting, can control blood sugar to a degree comparable to medication, while also helping you lose the excess weight that contributes to your insulin resistance. In addition, aerobic training—which refers to any exercise that keeps your heart rate up over a prolonged period of time—not only lowers your blood glucose, but also improves the circulation in your arms and legs (a common problem found in diabetics), rids you of stress, and helps you sleep better at night. A good exercise regimen consists of moderate physical activity performed three to five times per week for thirty minutes at a time.

As with a new diet, always talk to your doctor before starting an exercise routine. If the activity is too intense, it can sometimes release stress hormones that increase the glucose level in your blood, which would result in the need for a little extra insulin after a heavy work-out. If you are already living with diabetes, a close eye on your blood sugar is always prudent.

Lose Weight

Excess weight creates a vicious circle that perpetuates type 2 diabetes. The state of being overweight causes insulin resistance in your muscles and fat tissues, which in turn forces your system to secrete more insulin. Increased insulin in your blood makes you more overweight by encouraging your body to store fat, which raises your body's insulin resistance further, and so on.

The most important step you can take to lose weight is to maintain a healthful diet. That means eliminating many of the foods so common to North American dinner tables. Fast food, refined sugar and flour, and soft drinks are all hallmarks of an poor diet. Their empty calories put stress on your system and contribute to insulin resistance. Once you cut them out of your meal plan you will see positive changes in your weight. According to the American Diabetes Association, shedding 10 to 15 pounds can have tremendous health benefits, including lower blood sugar, reduced blood pressure, improved cholesterol levels, and less stress on your joints—not to mention the fact that you will find it easier to engage in physical activity, which can also help you lose weight.

Some of the most encouraging information comes from the National Health Institutes, which states that a healthy diet and exercise cut your risk of developing type 2 diabetes by 58 percent. Always discuss any potential weight-loss regimen with your doctor, particularly if you are already a diabetic, as your insulin, blood sugar, and any medications you are taking will need to be closely monitored.

Sleep

Although diet and exercise are very important elements in the achievement of a desirable body weight and normal blood sugar levels, sleep appears to be heavily involved in the equation, as well. Sleep deprivation has been linked to insulin resistance and even obesity, with research suggesting that people who get less than seven to eight hours of sleep per night show an increased risk of acquiring type 2 diabetes. If you are already a type 2 diabetic, of course, sleep should be an even bigger priority.

There appears to be a strong link between sleep and your body's control of glucose. An insufficient amount of sleep disrupts the normal regulation of blood sugar levels that occurs during the stages of rest. Sleep also helps you maintain an appropriate weight by increasing your body's production of the protein hormone *leptin*, which suppresses appetite, and decreasing production of the hormone *ghrelin*, which stimulates appetite. This may explain why people who get inadequate sleep are more likely to be overweight than those who get their rest.

Take Vitamin D$_3$

Thus far, much has been said about vitamin D$_3$'s potential to stop illnesses such as stroke, heart attacks, and cancer, and the story is no different here. Evidence suggests that adequate levels of vitamin D$_3$ can help you avoid type 2 diabetes and increase your life expectancy if you already have the disease.

In one study, it was shown that those with diabetes have a much lower level of vitamin D$_3$.[11] In another study, vitamin D$_3$ levels were linked to survival rates of patients suffering from a combination of heart disease, hypertension, type 2 diabetes, and renal failure. Those patients with the lowest levels of the nutrient had a one-year survival rate of 66 percent, while those with the highest levels had a one-year survival rate of 96 percent.[12]

Sufficient levels of vitamin D$_3$ have displayed the ability to improve insulin sensitivity, even in people whose blood sugar is normal.[13] Research suggests that vitamin D$_3$ also plays a role in proper insulin secretion through its protective effects on beta cells (the pancreatic cells that produce insulin).[14] Damage to beta cells is the reason diabetics still succumb to the ravages of the illness even when it is under "control" through other medications. It is due to this fact that the preservation of beta cells is paramount.

For anyone with a family history of type 2 diabetes, I recommend a daily vitamin D$_3$ dose of 2,000 IU. If you already have type 1 or type 2 diabetes, I suggest upping the dosage to 5,000 IU per day. If you have darker skin, your vitamin D$_3$ levels are generally going to be lower than the norm. In this case, you may need to double your daily dose. The best way to figure out how much vitamin D$_3$ you require is to have your blood levels tested and strive to raise them to between 50 and 80 ng/mL.

Consider Other Supplements

In addition to vitamin D$_3$, there are a number of other supplements that can help improve type 2 diabetes by encouraging the proper metabolism of glucose in your system. The following examples have shown the most promise.

Chromium

Chromium is an essential trace mineral required for proper metabolism of carbohydrates, fats, and proteins. It has also shown to promote increased glucose tolerance in type 2 diabetics.[17] Studies have shown that taking a daily chromium supplement of 1,000 mcg significantly improves glucose levels as well as HbA1c levels, the common indicator of type 2 diabetes.[18]

Cinnamon

Researchers have determined that cinnamon contributes to a healthy glucose metabolism. A study by the US Department of Agriculture discovered that cinnamon contains water soluble compounds called *polyphenol polymers,* which increase insulin-dependent glucose metabolism twenty fold.[19] These compounds essentially turn on insulin-receptor genes, thereby raising glucose uptake and lowering blood glucose levels.[20]

To take advantage of its potential, add at least $1/4$ to $1/2$ teaspoon of cinnamon twice a day to your diet. You can add it to toast, tea, coffee, oatmeal (cold cereals are not recommended at any time). You can also use supplement capsules called *Cinnulin PF.* Simply follow the directions on the bottle for dosage.

Coenzyme Q_{10}

A compound naturally produced in the body, coenzyme Q_{10}, or CoQ_{10}, improves blood sugar control, lowers blood pressure, and prevents oxidative stress caused by free radicals. Appropriately, individuals with high blood sugar and cholesterol are often found to be deficient in this compound. Thankfully, supplementation has shown positive results.

In human trials, type 2 diabetics who were given 100 mg of CoQ_{10} twice daily showed increased blood sugar control and blood pressure.[21] In another study, CoQ_{10} supplementation improved blood flow in type 2 diabetics, an outcome attributed to its ability to lower vascular oxidative stress.[22] Finally, in animal studies, CoQ_{10} has proven to neutralize free radicals, improve blood flow, lower triglyceride levels, and raise HDL cholesterol levels, which suggests that the compound may have a role in preventing and managing complications due to diabetes.[23]

I recommend 100 mg of CoQ$_{10}$ once to three times daily. Make certain you check with your healthcare provider before starting supplementation, of course.

Dehydroepiandrosterone

Dehydroepiandrosterone, or DHEA, is a naturally occurring hormone that is easily converted into testosterone and estrogen. It also improves insulin sensitivity in type 2 diabetics, who tend to have low levels of the hormone.[24,25] Although the mechanisms behind this improvement aren't fully understood, it has been suggested that DHEA's conversion to testosterone may be responsible, as testosterone raises insulin sensitivity.[26] Research into DHEA has also shown a potential benefit to type 1 diabetics, as DHEA seems to increase pancreatic beta cells—the cells that are responsible for making and secreting insulin—in animals.[27] Other advantages of DHEA supplementation include its ability to produce antioxidant enzymes in the liver, reduce fat tissue, relieve stress, strengthen the immune system, maintain sexual desire, and improve mental clarity.

The dosage of DHEA depends on a number of variables, including your height, weight, gender, and even your stress level. I recommend that women start with 25 mg per day, and men with 50 to 100 mg per day. Getting your DHEA-S level checked in advance will give you a sense of the amount of DHEA that would suit your body. Because DHEA can cause high levels of testosterone and estrogen in your body, however, anyone with a history of breast or prostate cancer should discuss the use of this compound with a doctor before beginning supplementation.

Fiber

Although it may not be the most exciting subject, the importance of fiber should not be understated. The profound effects that fiber can have on your body coupled with the ease with which it can be incorporated into your diet make it a powerful tool. The addition of high-fiber foods to your daily meals prevents and reduces the potential damage caused by type 2 diabetes by reducing blood glucose levels an average of 10 percent.[28] In addition, fiber is nutrient dense, improves digestion, and induces a sense of fullness after eating, which prevents you from overeating. When increasing fiber, however, you must do it slowly in order to avoid adverse affects that may include bloating, flatulence, and cramps.

Consider getting a total of 30 to 35 g of fiber daily, which can be found in foods such as fruit, vegetables, oat bran, oatmeal, dried beans, and sesame seeds. I also recommend eliminating any "white" foods from your meals, including white rice, pasta, bread, potatoes, and sugar. All of these foods quickly result in very high levels of insulin in your body. Over time, these elevated insulin levels can cause your cells to lose their insulin sensitivity.

Green Tea Extract

Green tea contains an abundant amount of *catechins*, which fall into the family of polyphenols previously discussed in connection with cinnamon. These compounds are powerful antioxidants that are particularly effective at ridding the pancreas and liver of toxins.[29] Animal studies have shown that the catechins found in green tea may play a role in the prevention of diabetes.[30] They have also shown an ability to stop the destruction of beta cells in rats.[31] Finally, lab studies suggest that green tea may suppress diet-induced obesity.[32]

I recommend adding 6 to 9 drops of green tea extract to 32 ounces of water and drinking the mixture throughout the day.

L-Carnitine

Biosynthesized mainly in the liver and kidneys, this compound has been shown to lower blood sugar, increase insulin sensitivity, optimize fat and carbohydrate metabolism,[15] and prevent cardiac nerve damage.[16] L-carnitine deficiency is common in type 2 diabetics, who would benefit from a supplement of 500 to 1,000 mg per day.

Lipoic Acid (Alpha-Lipoic Acid)

Lipoic acid is a potent antioxidant that helps prevent the heart and kidney damage that often accompanies diabetes.[33] It also reduces fat accumulation and protects pancreatic beta cells.[34] Dosage of alpha-lipoic acid to treat diabetes usually ranges from 100 to 200 mg taken three times a day. This supplement works best when used in combination with *gamma-linolenic acid,* or GLA—an omega-6 fatty acid found in plant-based oils. GLA should be taken at dosages of 400 to 600 mg per day.

SKRMs

Medical breakthroughs are occurring in an unexpected area: food. Medical foods are defined by the Food and Drug Administration as "prescribed by a physician when a patient has special nutrient needs in order to manage a disease or health condition, and the patient is under the physician's ongoing care." These foods are called *selective kinase receptor modulators,* or SKRMs (pronounced skirm), because they affect enzymes called *kinases,* which activate or inhibit various molecules, including proteins, fats, and carbohydrates. Up to 518 different kinases have been identified in humans.

With this in mind, researchers are in search of foods that can target and modulate selected kinases in an attempt to alter the course of diseases such as type 2 diabetes. Two of the most promising foods in this field are hops and acacia, which have actually been utilized medicinally in certain cultures for centuries. These plants have been shown to support healthy blood sugar and triglyceride levels, and thus may be recommended to patients who have been diagnosed with metabolic syndrome or type 2 diabetes.[35] Insinase, a nutritional supplement designed by the Metagenics company to improve glucose metabolism, contains both of these naturally occurring SKRMs. Talk to your healthcare provider to see if medical food supplements would benefit your situation.

CONCLUSION

Both type 1 and type 2 diabetes are progressive illnesses that slowly destroy your body, even when controlled by medication. Although there may be a possible connection between low levels of vitamin D$_3$ and type 1 diabetes, for now the disease remains a genetic mystery. Type 2, however, appears to be caused by a number of modifiable factors, including weight, exercise, and sleep, as well as vitamin D$_3$ intake.

Weight loss, regular physical activity, and sufficient rest all contribute to a decreased chance of acquiring type 2 diabetes, not to mention a possible reversal of its symptoms, should you already be affected by the illness. And all three of these treatments work best in concert, each boosting the effectiveness of the other. Exercise helps you lose weight and sleep better, while more sleep aids in weight loss, making it easier for you to exercise.

Additionally, by maintaining an adequate level of vitamin D$_3$, you can improve insulin sensitivity in your body, reduce excessive insulin production, and prevent the loss of vital pancreatic beta cells. Include a few of the supplements mentioned in this chapter to your daily routine and you will soon achieve a strong defense against type 2 diabetes. The most important thing to realize is that a diagnosis of this illness is not irreversible. If you pay attention to the signs of type 2 diabetes and make the right changes to your lifestyle early enough, you can bring your body back to normal and avoid the serious complications that usually follow this all-too-common disease.

8

Kidney Disease

I left the community of Spanish Harlem to join the United States Air Force when I was eighteen. After serving my country, I studied medicine, completing my training in obstetrics and gynecology at the University of Michigan. I subsequently moved to Texas with my family and remained there for twenty years. Forty-three years had passed before I decided to live in New York again. Upon my return, I met a childhood friend who told me of an upcoming reunion of the "old guys" from the neighborhood. I decided to check it out. When I got there, I was surprised at how different everyone looked. I didn't recognize most of them. Only when we began to exchange childhood stories did I realize who most of them were.

As a physician, one of the things that amazed me was how many of my old friends looked ill. It appeared as though almost every single person was suffering from one or more of the sicknesses discussed in this book. As I inquired into the health of each of my friends, my suspicions were confirmed. But they weren't the only ones affected—their sisters, brothers, parents, and extended family members all seemed to have fallen victim to disease. One guy—the neighborhood mechanical genius who had earned the nickname "the Professor" back in the day—told me that he had recently suffered kidney failure. As I began to write this chapter, I decided to call him and ask exactly what had happened.

Basically, he had let his high blood pressure run rampant for over thirty years. On occasion, his blood pressure had reached levels as high as 230/170. By the time he decided to take the condition seriously, it was too late. He had already entered into end-stage renal disease, which meant his kidneys were failing and would require dialysis while the search for an organ donor took place. This is where his story got even more disturbing.

During the search for a suitable kidney transplant donor, the first people tested as possible candidates are always members of the patient's family. Sadly, when the organ transplant agency looked into my ailing friend's family, it discovered that his sister, brother, and mother were all suffering from hypertension and had to be eliminated from consideration. Thankfully, an outside donor was eventually found.

I asked my friend how many medications he was taking. He counted twelve—some to prevent rejection of the transplant, others to prevent blood clots, and more to control his blood pressure. As we continued our discussion, I inquired about the other guys with whom we had grown up. He told me that at least three of them were in the middle of dealing with end-stage renal failure themselves, and that most of them were suffering from hypertension. Yet again, it appeared as though African Americans had become poster children for another deadly disease. After looking into the statistics, that suspicion was confirmed.

According to the National Kidney Foundation, black Americans are four times more likely to fall victim to kidney disease than white Americans. They also develop the condition at an earlier age than do white Americans, and suffer from end-stage renal disease approximately three times as often as white Americans. Although African Americans make up about 14 percent of the country's population, they account for 29 percent of kidney failure patients. Many of the risk factors of kidney disease include the other illnesses mentioned in this book. It is important to recognize the interconnectedness of the diseases that have come to plague our neighborhoods. By neglecting one illness, you may be allowing another to develop.

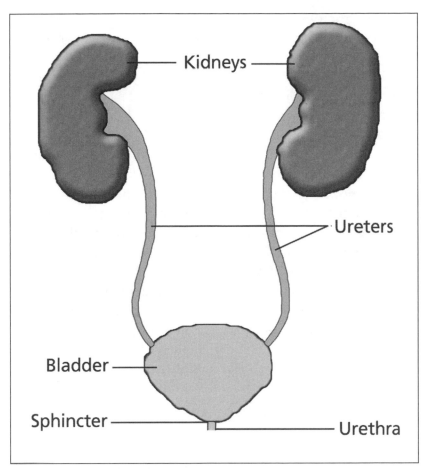

Figure 8.1. Image of Human Kidneys

WHAT IS KIDNEY DISEASE?

Located just below the middle of the back, one on either side of the spine, the kidneys perform numerous important functions in the body. (See Figure 8.1.) They help control your blood pressure, maintain your acid-base balance, regulate your levels of water and salt, and produce hormones such as *calcitriol* (vitamin D3), *renin* (part of the renin-angiotensin-aldosterone system mentioned earlier in the book), and *erythropoietin* (a necessary element in the creation of red blood cells). Perhaps their most well-known purpose is the filtration of blood and subsequent removal of residual waste, which makes its way to the bladder and gets excreted through urination.

Chronic kidney disease is characterized by a gradual decrease in kidney function, which causes a host of health problems, including the accumulation of waste in the body, high blood pressure, excess acid in the body (called *acidosis*), and anemia. After deteriorating over a number of years, the kidneys can eventually cease to work completely. Individuals whose kidneys have weakened to below 10 percent of their normal ability are considered "end-stage renal disease" patients. They require dialysis, which is the regular filtration of the blood by an external machine, or a replacement kidney from a donor.

Early symptoms of kidney disease include protein in the urine, swelling of the ankles and legs, frequent urination during the night, fatigue, itching, and high blood pressure. The illness is associated with a number of factors and conditions, some of which have been discussed in previous chapters of this book, including hypertension, diabetes, and even simply being African American.

WHAT CAUSES KIDNEY DISEASE?

The causes of kidney disease are many. While it can be inherited—as in the case of polycystic kidney disease—or derived from conditions of the immune system—as in the case of lupus—or brought about by other illnesses such as AIDS, hepatitis B, and hepatitis C—these causes are not the main culprits. The most common factors behind renal insufficiency, in fact, are diabetes and high blood pressure. This news is especially distressing for African Americans, who suffer from these illnesses in greater numbers than the general population. In addition, research is beginning to suggest a possible genetic predisposition towards end-stage renal disease in African Americans. Thankfully, there are ways to slow the damaging effects of these contributing factors and perhaps even avoid them entirely, of which you will be reminded later on in this chapter.

Diabetes

Just as high blood pressure can lead to kidney disease by over-working your blood vessels, so too can the high blood sugar levels caused by diabetes. In addition to damaging the filtration system of your kidneys, diabetes can have a destructive effect on nerves in your body, making it difficult for you to empty your bladder. This, in turn, promotes infection of the urinary tract, which can back up into your kidneys, injuring them. As previously mentioned, diabetes and hypertension are not only the two leading contributors to kidney disease but also signature illnesses of the black community. By finding ways to curb the prevalence of these conditions in our neighborhoods, we will also improve the health of our kidneys.

Drugs and Toxins

The prolonged overuse of painkillers such as acetaminophen (Tylenol), ibuprofen (Advil), and naproxen (Aleve) may result in injury to the kidneys by a process called *analgesic nephropathy,* another cause of kidney disease. The use of illegal intravenous drugs has also been connected to renal failure. Finally, kidney disease has been associated with environmental factors such as heavy metals, industrial chemicals, and viral infections.

Genetics

The rate of death from heart disease is 50 percent higher for black Americans than it is for white Americans, while the death rate from stroke is 80 percent higher for black Americans than it is for white Americans. These statistics, however, don't even come close to the prevalence of kidney failure in the black community. The rate of end-stage renal disease is an incredible 320 percent higher for black Americans than it is for white Americans.[1,2] Although kidney disease is associated with other health conditions common to the black community such as high blood pressure and diabetes, not to mention socioeconomic factors, these reasons alone do not account for the overwhelming prevalence of the illness in African

Americans.[3,4] In fact, some of the most interesting research suggests a genetic predisposition to the problem.

Scientists have linked the risk of kidney disease with the overexpression of a protein called *transforming growth factor beta 1*, or TGF-β1.[5] TGF-β1 is a protein that helps your body heal wounds by causing inflammation and scarring, both of which increase your risk of acquiring hypertension and kidney disease. Unfortunately, high levels of TGF-β1 can lead to an excess production of the fibrous connective tissue involved in scarring. Called *fibrosis*, this excess has been implicated in the above-average rates of hypertension and end-stage renal failure in the black community. Studies have shown that blacks with hypertension and end-stage renal disease have greater TGF-β1 levels than do whites with the same conditions.[6] It seems as though African Americans may simply be at a disadvantage due to naturally elevated levels of this important protein.

Combine this genetic predisposition to kidney disease with the occurrence of hypertension, diabetes, and socioeconomic stress, and you have a formula that explains the staggering death rate from end-stage renal disease in the black community.

Hypertension

Hypertension forces the heart to work harder, which damages blood vessels throughout the body, including those found in the kidneys. Over time, the gradual increase in blood pressure takes its toll on the kidneys, causing damage to their blood flow. This sets up a vicious circle of events. As the kidneys incur damage, they become less able to perform their necessary functions, which include waste removal, the regulation of the body's water levels, and the production of renin, the hormone that controls blood pressure. Of course, this simply creates a further elevation in blood pressure, which means more damage to the kidneys, and so on. There is an estimated 25,000 new cases of kidney failure caused by hypertension in the United States every year.[7]

Sadly, in the projects where I grew up, most people never knew about the importance of checking their blood pressure, and probably still don't realize it. Most, I suspect, don't understand that there is a cause-and-effect relationship between hypertension and kidney disease. This is unfortunate, as the occurrence of hypertension is generally higher in the population of the projects—a reality that is due, in part, to stress.

Obesity

As you already know, obesity plays a main role in type 2 diabetes and hypertension, both of which are major contributors to kidney failure. What you may not know is that obesity has been linked to end-stage renal disease independent of diabetes and high blood pressure. The heavier you are, the more work your kidneys have to do to keep your body functioning properly. Eventually, these organs just get worn out and fail.

HOW DO YOU REDUCE THE RISK OF KIDNEY DISEASE?

Although kidney disease may seem inevitable, the remarkable truth is that it is highly preventable—even for African Americans, who may have a genetic predisposition to kidney failure. By taking steps to control or avoid the conditions that contribute to renal insufficiency, you can overcome these potential problems. Nothing is written in stone. As many of the factors behind this debility are interrelated, treating one issue often helps treat another. That means controlling your blood pressure and blood sugar by using many of the same methods mentioned in previous chapters. By understanding how to maintain or improve your health through lifestyle changes and nutritional supplements, you may even be able to avoid traditional pharmaceuticals altogether. The following recommendations are intended not only to prevent or treat kidney disease but also to improve your overall health, which will have a protective effect against a number of illnesses.

Exercise

There is simply no substitute for physical activity when it comes to benefiting your long-term health. Exercise helps maintain proper blood sugar levels, alleviates high blood pressure, and fights obesity. In doing so, it reduces the burden placed on the kidneys by these conditions. Exercise also helps decrease stress, thereby eliminating the damaging compounds produced by stress. Thirty minutes of moderate physical activity a day—even if that activity merely consists of going for a walk—will do you a world of good.

Lose Weight

Losing weight is one of the best things you can do for your health. Shedding those extra pounds will improve kidney function by lightening the workload they are forced to bear every day. Of course, slimming down will also help you alleviate or even avoid the destructive tendencies of type 2 diabetes and high blood pressure, which constitute the two biggest causative factors of kidney disease. For example, research has shown that blood pressure begins to decline with a 10-percent loss of total body weight. Because a healthful body weight is good for your system in so many ways, its importance must not be underestimated or ignored.

Reduce Stress

Stress causes a rush of cortisol and norepinephrine in your system. These hormones raise your blood pressure, preparing you to either fight the stressor or flee from it. Although it is only a temporary reaction, the elevation in blood pressure can still damage blood vessels, which can lead to impaired kidney function.

While you may know about the importance of reducing your stress level, it is easier said than done. Steps you can take to decrease stress include exercise, breathing slowly, getting proper rest, meditation, and simplifying your life. One of the best stress reducers ever recorded, in fact, is prayer. You may also consider taking a supplement called *l-theanine.* L-theanine is an amino acid found in tea and Bay Bolete mushrooms that has been shown to reduce mental and physical stress while improving your cognition and mood.[8,9] It does so by increasing the level of a neurotransmitter called *gamma-aminobutyric acid,* which regulates your brain's excitatory response,[10] and dopamine, which enhances cognition. Single doses can range from 50 to 200 mg, with a maximum recommended daily amount of 1,200 mg.

Also mentioned in the chapter on diabetes, DHEA is a hormone that balances cortisol. As a result, supplements of this kind would be helpful during times of stress. I suggest that women take 25 mg per day and men take 50 mg per day.

Reduce Your Salt Intake

People with reduced kidney function also have an impaired ability to excrete salt. Excess salt in the body causes water retention, which increases blood pressure. Increased blood pressure further damages the kidneys, worsening their capacity to excrete salt. In this case, a low-salt diet is advised. Though the average American consumes far more than this amount, the recommended daily intake of salt for healthy individuals is 2,400 mg, or about 1 teaspoon. A low-salt diet would range from anywhere between 1,000 mg and 2,000 mg, depending on your condition. Using salt substitutes, some of which mix sea salt with herbs, is another option that can lower your overall salt intake. An easy method to monitor the amount of salt in your diet is to salt your food only after it has been prepared and not during cooking. That way, you can use as little as you please.

Finally, anyone dealing with kidney problems should follow the DASH diet, which was designed to lower high blood pressure. It involves eating mainly fruits, vegetables, legumes, and lean meats while also cutting down on fatty foods, sugar, and red meat. If you suffer from renal disease, controlling blood pressure is the most important thing you can do to combat further damage to your kidneys.

Take Vitamin D₃

As you learned in Chapter 4, vitamin D_3 has demonstrated the ability to lower blood pressure by preventing the overproduction of renin in the renin-angiotensin-aldosterone system, which, when found in excess, sets off a series of reactions that result in hypertension. In this manner, vitamin D_3 has a protective effect on the kidneys, fending off damage that can lead to or worsen kidney disease. In addition to this benefit, vitamin D_3 hinders the development of fibrosis, which, as previously mentioned, can sometimes occur during the healing process of an injured organ or tissue.[11] Finally, the nutrient counteracts the anemia that often results from chronic kidney disease.[12]

I recommend taking between 2,000 and 5,000 IU of vitamin D_3 per day as a protective measure, depending on your current blood levels of the nutrient.

Take Vitamin K_2

Vitamin K_2 can help you avoid the typical hardening of the arteries associated with kidney disease. It supports proper calcium metabolism, preventing calcium from being deposited in inappropriate places in your body, including your blood vessels. The recommended daily allowance of this nutrient is 80 mcg for men and 65 mcg for women, with infants requiring only 5 mcg. While it is possible to get your daily dose of vitamin K_2 from dietary sources such as leafy greens and vegetables, most people do not and would thus benefit from supplementation.

Consider Traditional Medication

Depending on the severity of your case and the effectiveness of the aforementioned therapies, you may have to rely on traditional medication to treat your kidney disease.

Patients are usually given a diuretic, also known as a water pill, as a first line of defense. Most commonly prescribed in the form of *hydrochlorothiazide,* a diuretic is one of the oldest means of inhibiting water retention and controlling the blood pressure of kidney disease and hypertension sufferers. Should this single medication not work, you may be asked to take an ACE inhibitor (angiotensin-converting enzyme inhibitor) or an ARB blocker (angiotensin receptor blocker) as well. As you know from chapter 4, ACE inhibitors reduce kidney damage by dilating blood vessels, while ARB blockers have a similar effect by preventing blood vessels from narrowing.

Other medications that alleviate high blood pressure and thus slow the destruction of the kidneys include beta-blockers, which decrease heart rate; calcium channel blockers, which relax muscles in the walls of blood vessels; vasodilators, which also relax blood vessel walls; and direct renin inhibitors, which suppress renin production, thereby stopping the RAAS from raising your blood pressure—exactly the same benefit that may be derived from vitamin D3 supplementation.

Ultimately, any medication has its pros and cons, all of which should be discussed with your doctor so that you can make an informed decision about your treatment.

CONCLUSION

The evidence is clear. Hypertension and diabetes are the two biggest risk factors for kidney disease. Neglecting to treat these with every method at your disposal can be disastrous to your well-being. Kidney disease affects your quality of life in every way imaginable once it has taken hold. It has both dire financial and emotional costs. These facts are especially alarming for African Americans, not only because they are more likely to suffer from hypertension and diabetes, but also because they are more likely to see these illnesses lead to fatal end-stage kidney disease. But do not despair. While statistics and even the recognition of a possible genetic predisposition should raise awareness of the problem, they should not extinguish hope. The prevention of renal illness and the alleviation of already established kidney problems can be achieved.

Your first line of defense includes watching your weight, maintaining a healthful diet (cutting down on salt, in particular), exercising, and reducing your stress level. Each of these lifestyle choices works against the damaging effects commonly caused by high blood pressure and diabetes, thus helping you avoid the destruction of your kidneys. In addition, as you have learned in previous chapters, incorporating a vitamin D_3 supplement into your health regimen is one of the best and easiest things you can do to fight renal failure. While vitamin D_3 can help lower the risk of kidney failure associated with hypertension and type 2 diabetes, it also appears to lessen some of the harmful symptoms of kidney disease, should you already be affected by the illness. Finally, traditional medication is available and should not be discounted. Lifestyle adjustments and nutritional supplements are powerful tools against kidney disease, but a doctor's prescription is never to be ignored. Always speak to your healthcare provider about all forms of treatment so that you may take full advantage of the options available to you.

9

Obesity

I t is estimated that up to 365 thousand deaths are caused by obesity in the United States every year.[1] Since 1980, the number of overweight children in this country has doubled while the number of overweight adolescents has tripled. But obesity is not confined to the United States. According to the World Health Organization, there are approximately 1 billion overweight adults worldwide, and 300 million of them are obese.

Obesity is a root cause of every one of the deadly illnesses mentioned in this book. Being overweight increases your body's workload, putting pressure on your heart and other organs, and thereby raising your risk of cardiovascular disease, kidney disease, and high blood sugar. The accumulation of fat results in inflammation and elevated hormone levels, both of which may lead to cancer.

Yet again, in comparison to the rest of the country, this problem affects African Americans disproportionately. According to the Office of Minority Health, African Americans are almost one and a half times as likely as white people to be obese. In particular, black women have a higher rate of obesity than any other group in the United States, with four out of five black women being overweight or obese. It is not, however, only adults who are affected by this issue. Statistics show that black children between the ages of six and seventeen years old are also more likely to be overweight than their white peers.

In general, obesity has reached epidemic proportions in this country and cannot be ignored if you wish to pursue a disease-free life. Sooner or later, it must be addressed and reversed in order for your body to be truly healthy.

WHAT IS OBESITY?

Technically speaking, there are two methods by which you can determine if you are overweight. The first involves measuring the circumference of your waist. The second involves measuring your body mass index, or BMI. Women are said to be at increased risk of poor health when their waistline measures 35 inches or greater, and men are said to be at risk when their waistline reaches 40 inches or more.

BMI indirectly determines your amount of body fat by assessing your weight relative to your height. To calculate your BMI, simply multiply your weight in pounds by 703, divide the result by your height in inches, and divide that result by your height in inches. The final value should fall somewhere in the range of numbers on the BMI scale, which have been categorized from "Underweight" all the way to "Obesity Class III." Table 9.1 outlines each category and the values associated with them.

TABLE 9.1. BMI CLASSIFICATIONS			
BMI	**Classification**	**BMI**	**Classification**
< 18.5	Underweight	30.0–34.9	Obesity Class I
18.5–24.9	Normal Weight	35.0–39.9	Obesity Class II
25.0–29.9	Overweight	> 40.0	Obesity Class III

Being overweight or obese simply means that your body has accumulated too much body fat. Body fat, also called *adipose tissue,* is essentially connective tissue whose primary purpose is to store energy. There are two types of adipose tissue: brown and white. Brown adipose tissue, or BAT, generates body heat and is found mostly in newborn human babies and hibernating mammals, which require it to keep warm. It is found only in very small amounts in adults. White adipose tissue, or WAT, is the body's major form of energy storage, and also acts as insulation and cushioning for the body and its organs. WAT makes up as much as 20 percent of a man's body mass and about 25 percent of a woman's.

Adipose tissue is also categorized according to location. Subcutaneous fat is located immediately under the skin. It cushions the body, contains nerves and blood vessels, and, of course, stores energy. Generally, it is not associated with the diseases related to obesity previously noted. Visceral fat is located inside the abdomen and around the internal organs. An excess of visceral fat most often results in enlarged midsections, commonly known as a "pot bellies," although researchers now suggest that even slim individuals can have an unhealthy amount of fat hidden in their abdomen if they get very little physical activity.

There is a direct link between visceral obesity and heart disease, hypertension, type 2 diabetes, as well as certain types of cancer.[2] An overabundance of fat cells promotes insulin resistance, which can lead to type 2 diabetes. Type 2 diabetes, as you now know, can lead to inflammation, hypertension, and kidney disease. Fat cells also disrupt your hormone levels. As discussed in Chapter 4, this disruption results in inflammation and high blood pressure. In addition, obesity places a tremendous strain on your heart muscle, which can eventually cause a heart attack. Finally, excess body fat can increase the production of a cancer-promoting estrogen called *estrone,* which, along with inflammation, may lead to a variety of cancers—particularly breast, prostate, uterine, and kidney cancer.

Because so many of these diseases are interconnected by this single factor, achieving or maintaining a healthful BMI is among the best things you can do for yourself. No other source makes this argument better than the famous Framingham Heart Study. According to its findings, lifespan decreases as BMI increases.[3] By analyzing groups of non-smokers, the study demonstrated that being overweight shortened the lives of women by 3.3 years and men by 3.1 years. The life expectancy of women who were categorized as Obesity Class I was reduced by 7.1 years, while the life expectancy of men in the same classification was cut by 5.8 years. Finally, women who fell into the category of Obesity Class III lost 8 years of their projected lifespan, while Obesity Class III men lost 13 years. Conversely, research shows that people who have a BMI of approximately 22.6—which is 15 percent below the national average—typically have the longest lifespan.

WHAT CAUSES OBESITY?

The simple cause of obesity is an increase in the consumption of high-calorie foods combined with a decrease in physical activity. In other words, you eat more than your body burns, and your body stores the excess as fat. But obesity is actually a little more complicated than that. While low energy expenditure certainly has a lot to do with weight gain, there are other factors that play a role in being overweight, including stress, poor thyroid function, and environmental toxins. In addition, obesity seems to display a cultural basis and possibly even a link to vitamin D_3 deficiency, which could explain the overrepresentation of African Americans in the rising rates of obesity in this country.

High-Calorie Diet and Lack of Physical Activity

Your body has minimum energy requirements to function properly. The number of calories required to maintain the physiological processes of a non-active human body is referred to as *resting energy expenditure*, or REE. The energy needs of your various organs account for about 70 percent of that number, with 20 percent used for non-exercise-related physical activity and the remaining 10 percent used to generate body heat.[4] When you take in more calories than dictated by your daily caloric requirement without also raising your energy level through physical activity, the excess calories are stored as fat, thus resulting in weight gain and possible future obesity. Of all the reasons behind weight gain, this one is certainly the most clear-cut.

Lack of exercise is actually a double-edged sword. It first promotes the formation of fat, which then has an effect on the hormones that regulate appetite. Research has shown that the appetite-suppressing hormone *leptin* is raised in obese individuals. While this information may seem contrary to common sense, scientists suspect that the elevated leptin may indicate obesity-induced leptin resistance, similar to the insulin resistance caused by prolonged high blood sugar levels, as discussed in Chapter 7. Thus, an obese person's hunger may not be satisfied quite as easily as the hunger of a slimmer person. In other words, weight begets weight.

Stress

The human body reacts to perceived threats by secreting hormones such as cortisol as part of the natural fight or flight response. In short bursts, this hormone is beneficial, providing energy, increased immunity, and heightened memory. Unfortunately, prolonged periods of raised cortisol activity are very destructive, resulting in high blood pressure, lowered immunity, and impaired cognitive function. They can also cause unintended weight gain.

When the body becomes stressed, cortisol causes glucose to be released into the bloodstream as a quick source of energy. Centuries ago, this energy would have come in handy to our ancestors, who would have needed the extra strength to avoid or battle a predator. In modern humans, however, whose sources of stress do not generally require such a response, this glucose goes unused and is eventually stored as fat. Cortisol also creates an imbalance between the aforementioned hormone leptin and the hormone *ghrelin,* as well as the amino acid *neuropeptide Y,* all of which regulate appetite.[5] This imbalance stimulates hunger and encourages energy to be stored as fat.[6] When stress becomes chronic, it can easily contribute to abdominal obesity.

Environmental Toxins

Although they have been linked to many other health issues, environmental toxins have rarely been mentioned in relation to weight gain. Chemical pollutants, however, can affect the regulation of weight in a number of ways. From the pesticides used in food production to the chemicals used by the plastics industry such as phthalates and bisphenol A, harmful synthetic substances find their way into the human body every day, slowly altering its ability to function properly. These toxins can cause inflammation, provoke the body's stress response, damage thyroid operation, promote insulin resistance, and impair metabolism, all of which lead to obesity.

In fact, protecting yourself isn't the only issue. Fetal exposure is of particular concern. There is now evidence that the environmental chemicals absorbed by a mother during pregnancy negatively affect her baby's birth weight and physiological function, and also promote gene malformation.[7] In addition to being possible carcinogens, both phthalates and the toxins found in cigarettes can disrupt the normal hormonal development of a fetus, contributing to childhood obesity.[8,9,10] Sadly, there are more chemicals found in babies than can be mentioned here. In fact, a study performed by the Environmental Working Group noted the presence of 287 toxins in the umbilical cord blood of a sample of newborns.[11] If you are pregnant, I recommend limiting your exposure to toxins as much as you can. Buying organic food and cutting out cigarette use can protect not only your health but also the health of your child.

Society and Culture

The African American Collaborative Obesity Research Network, or AACORN, estimates that at least 86 percent of black women will be overweight by the year 2015, while 62 percent will be obese.[12] Although certain physiological differences may play a role in the rate of obesity in black Americans, society and culture appear to play even bigger roles.

According to AACORN, there are multiple factors that contribute to the high obesity levels in black neighborhoods. These include a lack of access to fresh fruit and vegetables, fewer facilities that offer physical activities, and an abundance of fast food restaurants. Particularly in children, socioeconomic deprivation seems to be a predictor of future obesity.

Being overweight is associated not only with social factors but with cultural ones as well. First, black Americans are more accepting of being overweight and obese. Second, black families, in general, do not place a high priority on nutrition in their daily meals, and this tradition is silently passed down the generations. While it may be delicious, most African American cuisine, or "soul food," is high in salt, fat, cholesterol, and calories.[13] Although these habits are hard to break, regularly eating in this manner is sure to result in significant weight gain.

Hypothyroidism

Located in the neck, the thyroid gland is responsible for producing hormones that regulate the body's metabolism. Hypothyroidism, or underactive thyroid gland, can cause fatigue, dry skin, poor memory, and weight gain. Since the symptoms are seemingly unrelated, hypothyroidism often goes undiagnosed for years. If you suspect that you may be suffering from this illness or have a family history of hypothyroidism, discuss it with your doctor, who can test your thyroid function. The problem can be effectively treated with medication.

Vitamin D₃ Deficiency

In a study published in the *Journal of Clinical Endocrinology & Metabolism*, insufficient vitamin D_3 was associated with stunted growth and increased weight in pubescent girls.[14] In another study, low levels of vitamin D_3 were linked to elevated weight, increased body mass index, and a greater occurrence of type 2 diabetes.[15] This research reflects the growing evidence for a strong relationship between low levels of vitamin D_3 and weight. Furthermore, this relationship seems to begin at an early age.

HOW DO YOU REDUCE THE RISK OF OBESITY?

While obesity is a major contributor to the onset of numerous diseases, it is also one of the most preventable risk factors for illness imaginable. For example, one study of hypertension and obesity suggests that the incidence of hypertension would decline by 48 percent in white individuals and 28 percent in black individuals if only their weight was properly controlled.[16]

By now you may be asking, "How do I lose weight?" Well, first and foremost, you have to watch your diet and engage in some physical activity. While a simple diet that is low in processed

Weight-Loss Drugs

I believe that weight-loss medications are dangerous and do not recommend them. Additionally, these drugs work only while you're taking them and do not solve the primary causes behind your weight gain. The most common diet pill is phentermine, which is part of the amphetamine family of drugs. Several years ago, phentermine was one of two drugs that were combined to form the anti-obesity medication fen-phen, which resulted in a number of deaths due to side effects such as primary pulmonary hypertension and heart valve problems. It has since been removed from the market.

It has been suggested that phentermine alone can cause the same problems. Furthermore, it has been associated with other harmful side effects, including increased heart rate, elevated blood pressure, and dependence. If you are a diabetic on insulin, there are special precautions that you must take before using phentermine, such as lowering insulin dosage accordingly.

Most healthcare providers will request an EKG and ask that you undergo a complete physical exam before considering phentermine as a weight-loss treatment. This medication is not recommended for those with pre-existing heart conditions, glaucoma, an overactive thyroid gland, or a history of drug abuse. In light of all these facts, pharmaceuticals, in my opinion, are not the answer to the problem of obesity.

sugar and fat but high in fruit and vegetables should generally help bring your weight to an ideal level, I understand that some of you will want to follow a more formal diet program in an attempt to shed your extra pounds. With that in mind, some of the more popular diet plans are discussed below.

In order to lose weight, sometimes you must consider more than just the typical reasons behind weight gain. Obesity may also be connected to factors such as stress, fatigue, or even environmental toxins. In those cases, you may benefit from vitamin D3 and other nutritional supplements, or simply more sleep. By taking the time to evaluate your own body and lifestyle, you will be able to determine the best course of action and follow your own personal weight-loss plan.

Change Your Diet

It takes 3,500 calories to make one pound of fat. Whether you decide to follow an established weight-loss plan or manage your weight on your own, it is this simple fact that will be the basis of your daily routine. Once you've determined what your daily caloric intake should be according to your height, age, and level of physical activity (there are many websites that can calculate it for you), you can begin to reduce your daily calorie count, knowing that every time you reach a reduction of 3,500 calories one pound of fat will be lost. For example, if you want to lose one pound per week, you'll need to cut 500 calories each day. Should that feel too severe, you can modify your plan to a more comfortable level. A daily reduction of 250 calories, which would result in the loss of one pound every two weeks, may be a more reasonable goal for you.

Many people choose a recognized weight-loss regimen to help them drop those unwanted pounds, but which one should you choose? Unfortunately, there are so many different diets that claim all sorts of amazing things that it is often difficult to sort fact from fiction. The truth is that the best diet is the one that works for you.

While low-fat diets can be effective, they can also lead to additional weight gain when the dieter focuses too much on cutting out fat and disregards calories. Too many calories from any source—even a low-fat one—will create extra pounds. In recent years, low-carb diets have been all the rage, helping people shed weight quickly. But studies have shown this method to be no more effective than a low-fat diet after about six months, and tough to maintain on a long-term basis. Its heavy reliance on protein and meat products can also be quite unhealthy. Glycemic-index diets rank foods according to their effect on blood sugar and are similar to the low-carb method, though the many factors that must be considered at every meal (your age, weight, how the food is prepared, portion size) can be daunting.

Meal-replacement diets, such as Slim-Fast, can work just as well as any other program. Each meal substitution provides less than 400 calories and is nutritionally complete. Replacing breakfast, or breakfast and lunch, with a low-calorie shake or meal bar can be quite effective when combined with a nutritious dinner of 600 to 700 calories. Meal providers, such as Jenny Craig, can also help, though they can be quite pricey. Perhaps the most encouraging results come from group programs, such as Weight Watchers. Studies have shown that the likelihood of success doubles when a dieter is a member of a group or clinic.[17]

Research shows that eight out of ten dieters are unable to maintain their weight loss for an extended period of time.[18] Perhaps this is because the dieters never really understood the reason behind their weight gain in the first place. Fad diets may be very successful initially, but if you don't realize the complex reasons behind your weight problem, you'll forever be yo-yo dieting, which is both depressing and unhealthy. Established diet methods can get you started in your battle against obesity, but ultimately, you will need to take a closer look at your overall way of life in order to control your weight.

The Culture of Obesity

Sometimes your cultural background can do a disservice to your health. This is certainly the case in the African-American community. The fatty, salty, and simply unhealthy cooking methods involved in "soul food" are proving to be a giant stumbling block for African Americans who want to lose weight. But you need not abandon your traditions outright. The same foods that have been giving you comfort over the years can be prepared in a healthier manner.[19] Instead of deep-frying your vegetables, sauté them in a low-sodium broth. Instead of bacon grease and butter, use olive or canola oil for cooking. Perhaps most importantly, taste your food before you add salt or butter for flavor. Small adjustments to your favorite meals can make a world of difference to your waistline and your general health.

Drink More Water

Water is an often overlooked tool in the fight against obesity. By increasing your water intake by about 16 ounces per day, you will boost your metabolic rate by 30 percent.[20] The consumption of eight 8-ounce glasses of water per day burns about 70 calories, while dehydration actually slows down fat metabolism. Water is also required to flush the toxins released by weight loss from your body. Finally, drinking water with a meal helps you lose weight by making you feel full sooner, which causes you to eat less.

Most experts recommend eight 8-ounce glasses of water per day. You may feel the need to drink a few glasses more, though, depending on your weight and level of physical activity.

Exercise

It goes without saying that exercise helps you lose weight. Even a brisk walk taken three or four times a week can be beneficial, especially if you are obese. Exercising alone, however, is not as effective as the combination of moderate exercise and a healthful diet.

Get More Sleep

Studies conducted at the New York University School of Medicine have revealed that a lack of sleep can have a profound effect on hormones. Sleep disturbances can significantly decrease levels of the appetite-suppressant leptin and raise levels of the appetite-stimulant ghrelin.[21,22,23] These studies have also shown a connection between increased appetite and an elevated consumption of calorie-dense foods. Fortunately, just as sleep deprivation can contribute to weight gain, the treatment of sleep disorders contributes to both weight loss and increased energy. To benefit from sleep, aim to get seven to eight hours of rest per night.

Take Vitamin D₃

It seems that there is a great deal of information available about vitamin D_3 as it relates to the prevention or alleviation of diseases such as type 2 diabetes, kidney disease, and cardiovascular disease, but very little direct evidence suggesting a relationship between the sunshine vitamin and obesity. Recently, however, a promising study conducted at the University of Minnesota demonstrated a connection between the two. Vitamin D_3 levels were monitored in thirty-eight overweight men and women before an eleven-week diet plan. All the subjects were deficient in vitamin D_3 at the study's outset. At the end of the eleven weeks, vitamin D_3 levels proved reliable predictors of weight loss success. When the subjects' vitamin D_3 levels rose, so did the amount of weight they lost. In addition, higher levels of vitamin D_3 were associated with a greater loss of dangerous visceral fat, which surrounds the organs in the abdomen.[24] Whether low vitamin D_3 levels are a causative factor in obesity or simply a by-product of it, it appears that vitamin D_3 supplementation can be of aid when you're trying to lose weight.

Consider Other Supplements

While a poor diet and lack of exercise are the two most obvious causes of obesity, other problems can play a part in weight gain. Factors such as stress, fatigue, and toxins can all wreak havoc on your system and raise your risk of being overweight. Fortunately, you can treat these issues with the help of nutritional supplements.

Coenzyme Q$_{10}$

Coenzyme Q$_{10}$ is a co-essential enzyme that can improve metabolism and boost energy levels. I recommended taking at least 100 mg per day, though that dosage may be taken up to three times per day, especially if you're on statin medications or have been diagnosed with chronic fatigue syndrome.

Glisodin

Glisodin is a powerful antioxidant that reduces the destructive free radical known as the reactive oxygen species while increasing energy production and minimizing fatigue. The supplement is derived from cantaloupe extract and a wheat protein. I recommend taking 150 mg once or twice a day, depending on your particular need.

Greens Powder

A concentrated powdered form of nutrient-dense foods such as wheatgrass, kale, chlorella, and spirulina, greens powder is packed with healthful compounds called *phytonutrients*. Greens not only provide nutrition but also alkalize your body, reducing the absorption of toxins and increasing the elimination of waste from your gastrointestinal tract. Read the manufacturer's instructions for dosage guidelines.

Green Tea Extract

Green tea extract is known to improve metabolism, increase fat burning, and support weight reduction. This ability is most likely a result of the combination of green tea's natural caffeine and catechins, the latter of which also has benefits for type 2 diabetics, as discussed in Chapter 7. Research shows that the consumption of green tea catechins along with exercise helps reduce visceral fat.[25] I recommend adding 6 to 9 drops of green tea extract to 32 ounces of water and drinking that mixture throughout the day.

Irvingia Gabonensis

Fiber can be a powerful addition to your weight loss plan. Fiber stays in your stomach longer, slowing your digestion and making you feel full for long periods of time. It also moves fat through your digestive tract quickly so that your body absorbs less of it. The extract of the Irvingia gabonensis seed is a fiber that has proven to be a particularly effective as a weight-loss supplement. The benefits of this supplement can be achieved by taking doses of 150 mg twice daily.

L-Carnitine

L-carnitine is an amino acid that is responsible for bringing fat to the mitochondria in your cells, which burn that fat as fuel for your body. Doses of 2 to 3 g per day are usually recommended as an aid in weight loss.

L-Theanine

As noted in Chapter 8, l-theanine is an amino acid found in tea and Bay Bolete mushrooms. It assists in managing stress and helps blunt the effects of cortisol. It also supports increased cognition and relaxation without causing drowsiness. I recommend taking 100 mg of l-theanine three times a day.

Reds Powder

Made largely from powdered fruit, reds powder provides similar detoxifying properties as green powder, along with the antioxidant protection of colorful foods such as raspberries, blueberries, cranberries, and pomegranates. Read the manufacturer's instructions for dosage guidelines.

Saffron

Saffron combats the emotional aspect of overeating by increasing serotonin levels in your body. Serotonin promotes a feeling of fullness while also alleviating stress and the onset of depression, all of which contribute to compulsive eating. Research has found that 30 mg taken twice daily can have a positive effect on weight loss.

5-Hydroxytryptophan

Also known as 5-HTP, this amino acid is involved in the conversion of tryptophan to serotonin, a neurotransmitter responsible for mood regulation. Studies have shown 5-HTP to be beneficial in the treatment of depression, anxiety, and even obesity-related binge eating, perhaps due to its connection to serotonin, which is a neurotransmitter responsible for mood regulation. 50 mg of 5-HTP taken two to three times a day can provide these benefits, but this supplement is not recommended if you are already taking other medications that increase serotonin levels, such as SSRIs.

CONCLUSION

As you now know, the problem of obesity is not quite as simple as it seems. While its basis lies in too many calories and too little energy expenditure, there are many other factors that can have an impact on your weight. These factors must be considered when embarking on a weight-loss routine. Failure to recognize obesity as a complex disease usually prevents an individual from achieving or maintaining weight loss. Without shedding a few pounds, however, overweight people face a long list of possible consequences, including type 2 diabetes, hypertension, kidney failure, liver problems, and even cancer.

In order to overcome a weight problem, you must not blindly choose a brand-name diet program or commercial product, but rather use the information provided in this chapter to determine its root cause. Once you've done that, you will be better able to figure out which type of plan is best for you. But regardless of your decision, at some point, exercise must become part of your daily regimen.

Note that I said "at some point." Some people are too easily fatigued due to obesity to start exercising at the beginning of their weight-loss campaign. In this case, I advise you to lose 5 to 7 pounds through diet alone and then try exercising. Losing even a small amount of weight will provide emotional encouragement and help restore the energy you need to exercise. Trying to exercise when you're not ready can cause stress, which raises the amount of cortisol in your system, ironically causing weight gain.

Along with exercise and proper nutrition, always make certain you maintain healthful vitamin D_3 levels, take whichever supplements might help you on your journey, drink plenty of water, and get your sleep. These elements are each an integral part of conquering obesity.

10

A Guide to Dietary Supplements

Choosing a nutritional supplement is intimidating. In recent years, the number and variety of supplements on store shelves have exploded, making the process of purchasing the right product for you even more confusing. But a trip to the supplements aisle doesn't have to be frustrating. This chapter provides a few brief but informative guidelines on purchasing and using dietary supplements that will help you hone in on the best products for your personal health plan.

WHOLE FOOD-BASED SUPPLEMENTS

Whenever possible, buy whole food-based supplements. Synthetic vitamins and minerals lack the complementary elements inherent to real food that help your body recognize and use each nutrient properly. When your body does not recognize the substance, it generally eliminates or stores it, making the supplement useless at best or potentially toxic at worst. Whole food-based supplements, on the other hand, are sourced from actual food and therefore contain numerous additional compounds that support bioavailability—which simply means they are easily absorbed by your body. While it may not be an option for every healthful supplement suggested by this book, choosing whole food-based products is always an important consideration. Finally, whether the supplement is whole food-based or not, always read the label on the bottle to determine if the product contains any ingredients that may cause an allergic reaction, such as soy, dairy, or gluten.

PROCESSING AND PACKAGING

The manner in which supplements are both processed and packaged has a significant effect on their nutritional impact. In the same way that overcooking a food destroys its nutrients, the strength of a supplement is diminished if it is heated beyond 125°F during processing. Whenever possible, look for a supplement that has been freeze-dried or processed at a low temperature. In addition to the effect of heat on supplements, exposure to light and air also diminishes their effectiveness. Dark plastic bottles do a better job of blocking light than do the typical white plastic bottles, but dark amber or dark blue glass bottles are the best choice. Also, always check that the bottle has been vacuum-sealed, which not only ensures that the product is fresh but also prevents anyone from tampering with its contents.

DOSAGE

You may be wondering why dosages for some of the supplements listed in this book are higher than the daily amounts recommended by the Food and Drug Administration. The answer is that the FDA's recommendations are merely designed to ward off conditions caused by nutritional insufficiencies. They are not intended to prevent or alleviate the diseases plaguing our modern lives. For example, a dose of 60 mg of vitamin C per day, as suggested by the FDA, will help you avoid scurvy, an illness caused by vitamin C deficiency. It will not, however, decrease your risk of cardiovascular disease, which, according to some studies, may be lowered by taking 300 mg of vitamin C per day. Similarly, while the FDA urges people to get 400 IU of vitamin D every day, diabetics have a much better chance of improving their insulin sensitivity by taking between 2,000 and 5,000 IU on a daily basis, to name but one of the positive effects of elevated vitamin D dosage.

In many instances, the FDA's recommendations are appropriate, and you should always be careful not to take any supplement in an amount that might result in toxicity. More and more, however, research is proving the advantages of exceeding the typical dosage of certain supplements. While this book provides you with detailed information on supplement quantities, you can always speak to your doctor for further advice on the subject.

TAKE ONLY WHAT YOU NEED

Once you have realized the benefits of dietary supplements, you may find yourself becoming a victim of marketing, wanting to buy every supplement that seems helpful. Unfortunately, I have seen this happen with many of my patients. The truth is that you probably don't need to buy everything on your local vitamin store's shelf. I recommend you start your plan with a basic multivitamin that has been designed specifically for your gender. Once you've chosen that, purchase the supplements that will help treat any chronic health conditions that may be affecting you. For example, you could use DHA capsules to treat your chronic inflammation. Lastly, if you feel any short-term health issues coming on, such as a cold, simply use the supplements that will alleviate it, and then discontinue use of those products. There is no reason to overdo supplementation. Listen closely to your body and take only what it truly needs.

CONCLUSION

Now that you are familiar with the kind of supplements to look for when you're shopping, you may be wondering where to shop. Your average drug store or grocery store should have a section for vitamins and other supplements, but the selection is usually small and typically made up of mostly synthetic products. Your best bet is to browse your local health food store, which generally has a wider array of options that includes numerous naturally derived supplements. Although the variety found at these stores can be intimidating, a number of my favorite products are listed in the Supplement Guidelines section (page 123) at the end of this book to help you make your choice. As long as you remember the guidelines set forth in this chapter, you will be on your way back home and enjoying the benefits of supplementation in no time.

Conclusion

When it comes to the health of the African-American community, you must ask yourself two questions: "How did we get here?" and "Where do we go from here?" If you hope to improve your health and increase your longevity, you must first determine how the rates of disease in the black community have reached such disturbing levels. How did we allow ourselves to have our health compromised to the extent that any of the diseases mentioned in this book invaded our households? It is a hard question to face, but it must be addressed. Once you have identified the factors that contribute to illness, you can then take advantage of every preventative measure available to you. Although you may not know it, these measures are all practical and achievable. You can enjoy your time on this planet and, most importantly, stop this plague of sickness from destroying another generation of black Americans. You must take action not only for your benefit but also for the good of the children. It is your responsibility to pass on everything you have learned from this book to the next group of young people, who need to be told about the positive effects that diet, lifestyle habits, and powerful disease-fighting substances such as vitamin D_3 can have on their well-being. If you don't get in their corner, who will?

HOW DID WE GET HERE?

As you now know, many factors, from poor nutrition to vitamin D_3 deficiency, have contributed to the present state of African-American health. But one cause that has not been adequately pointed out is the failure of the medical establishment to raise awareness of existing solutions in the black community.

As much as I would like to criticize pharmaceutical companies harshly for dropping the ball here, I suppose it is not their responsibility to promote anything other than that which improves their bottom line and compensates their stockholders. It is naïve to think that any pharmaceutical company would advertise a supplement such as vitamin D_3, which, due to its inexpensive nature, might adversely affect future profits.

But what about doctors? Shouldn't they be championing the ideas set forth in this book? Well, the truth is that most doctors are not very knowledgeable about the use of vitamins and supplements as a means of preventing or treating disease. Perhaps due to a lack of time, or maybe because medical schools do not embrace non-traditional methods easily, the subject just isn't a big part of a doctor's training. Furthermore, don't think for a minute that pharmaceutical companies don't exert an influence on medical students. They supply lunches at clinics, hire speakers for seminars, and pay for much of the research performed at these institutions. Unfortunately, they advocate disease management, not prevention. Prevention is an infrequent part of medical training—except for what we doctors call primary prevention, which is basically telling people to get their immunizations, pap smears, and breast exams, to name a few examples. Doctors in training learn to treat an illness, but typically only with traditional drugs. Although a doctor may consider expanding his scope of expertise after graduating from medical school, debt from student loans combined with the years spent waiting to officially *be* a doctor often cause him to stick to what he knows and get to work. It is upsetting that the African-American community has been let down by modern medical practices for so many years, but things change, and thankfully, I can say that I am not the only one endorsing an alternative mindset these days. Doctors all over the country have begun to think outside the box.

WHERE DO WE GO FROM HERE?

Diet, exercise, and nutritional supplementation are all lifestyle decisions that you can make as an adult in charge of your own destiny. But if you are truly concerned about improving the longevity of your family, helping the unborn and the newly born is paramount. To lower the rates of illness in the next generation, you can take steps to ensure that children are made stronger and more resilient—a process that starts even before conception.

Vitamin D₃ and Pregnancy

Health and longevity begin even before you are born. Pregnancy is a time when huge strides can be taken towards a child's well-being. In particular, proper vitamin D_3 levels during pregnancy have been associated with a lower chance of premature delivery, an increase in the baby's birth weight, and an improvement in infant bone strength. They may also reduce the risk of schizophrenia, brain tumors, asthma, multiple sclerosis, and type 1 diabetes.[1]

The current recommended daily dose of vitamin D_3 for pregnant women is 400 IU, which is actually a very low amount according to all the latest research on the subject. The American Academy of Pediatrics has stated that prenatal vitamins containing 400 IU of vitamin D_3 have little effect on circulating maternal vitamin D levels, and have declared such a dosage inadequate for pregnant women.[2] In agreement with this statement, The Canadian Pediatric Society strongly suggests a dosage of 2,000 IU, especially for winter pregnancies. And while vitamin D may be found in food sources such as cod liver oil and fortified milk, when vitamin D-producing sunlight is not in abundance, it is almost impossible to reach the optimal amount of this nutrient without supplementation.

Finally, breastfed babies should receive their own supplemental vitamin D_3 within two months of being born. Although breast milk is the best form of nourishment for a baby, it nevertheless lacks a sufficient amount of vitamin D. Vitamin D deficiency is even more likely in breastfed babies who do not get enough sunlight. The American Academy of Pediatrics recommends 400 IU of vitamin D_3 per day for all infants, whether taken as a supplement, in the case of breastfed babies, or acquired from formula, in the case of bottle-fed babies.

DHA and Pregnancy

In addition to vitamin D_3, *docosahexaenoic acid*, or DHA, has proven to be very beneficial to the brain and eye development of an unborn child. DHA is an omega-3 fatty acid, which is most abundantly found in oily fish but can be taken as a supplement instead. While omega-3 fatty acids also come in a form called *eicosapentaenoic acid*, or EPA, it is the DHA form that has proven particularly important during pregnancy.

The consumption of DHA supplements is associated with better attention spans in babies up to six months of age, better visual learning at one year and eighteen months of age, as well as improved language skills.[3] DHA intake during pregnancy has been connected to higher IQ scores in children up to four years of age, good sleep patterns, reduced allergies, increased birth weight, and a lower chance of premature delivery.[4,5,6,7] In addition to helping the fetus, DHA also helps the mother by decreasing her risk of postpartum depression.[8]

Although fish is the best source of omega-3s, the mercury content of many fish is a huge concern for pregnant women. While the FDA recommends 12 ounces of cooked fish per week for pregnant women, it advises against the consumption of large predatory fish such as shark, swordfish, and mackerel, as these varieties contain higher concentrations of mercury.[9,10] Fish that have lower amounts of mercury include salmon, pollock, and shrimp, but no species is completely free of the toxic substance.

Flaxseed has been touted as an alternative source of omega-3 fatty acids, as it converts a compound called *alpha-linolenic acid*, or ALA, into DHA. The rate of conversion, however, is extremely inefficient, resulting in very little DHA. More importantly, the consumption of flaxseeds during pregnancy may actually be harmful, having been linked to birth defects and spontaneous abortions in some studies.[11]

The easiest way to ensure your DHA intake is through supplements. The majority of DHA supplements are essentially fish oil capsules, so you must still be vigilant about the source of the oil and the manner in which it is processed, which affect its mercury content. For those who wish to avoid fish altogether, there are vegetarian DHA supplements available, which are derived from algae. A dosage of 1,000 mg of DHA per day can provide numerous benefits to your unborn child.

Folic Acid and Pregnancy

The importance of folic acid—also known as vitamin B_9—during pregnancy has been well established. Folic acid deficiency can result in neural tube defects in a growing fetus, including the incomplete closure of the spinal cord and spinal column known as *spina bifida*, and the severe underdevelopment of the brain known as *anencephaly*. Future mothers should take every opportunity to avoid these possible outcomes. Due to red blood cell synthesis and nutritional demands of the unborn child, a mother's stores of this vitamin steadily decline throughout gestation.[12] While many foods are fortified with vitamin B_9, women are advised to take a daily B complex vitamin (folic acid is better absorbed in combination with the other B vitamins) throughout pregnancy as a precaution. Neural tube defects associated with low folic acid can be all but eliminated by taking between 600 and 800 mcg of the vitamin daily. In fact, women should begin supplementation at least one month before attempting to conceive in order to ensure good folic acid levels during the first month of pregnancy, when a deficiency can be extremely detrimental to proper fetal growth.[13,14,15]

AFRICAN-AMERICAN HEALTHY

You should now have a good understanding of the illnesses that have been plaguing African Americans for years. Hypertension, cancer, stroke, type 2 diabetes, kidney disease, and obesity have each become a big part of the black experience, diminishing quality of life and frequently ending life itself. It is clear that the high rates of disease in the black community are connected to a wide variety of factors, including diet, exercise, and even genetics. It is also clear that a great number of these factors can be addressed to help you avoid getting sick. If you start to pay attention to the types of food you eat and your level of physical activity, you can make great strides towards living a disease-free life. In addition, by learning about your specific physiology as an African American, you will finally understand how to bring your system to its optimum state.

African Americans as a people seem to be prone to certain detrimental biological conditions, including vitamin D deficiency, elevated TGF-β1, and even increased stress, all of which raise the chance of acquiring disease. Fortunately, there are a number of different supplements available that can help you alleviate these predispositions and put you on an equal footing with the rest of the country. You do not have to simply "get by," dependent on expensive pharmaceuticals for the rest of your days. By changing your perspective on health, you will change your life. Once you have changed your life, you must take steps to change your neighborhood. Spread the word so that the next generation, and every generation to come, will have a different outlook on what it means to grow up black. Give the children better expectations than you had, and help them meet those expectations. By becoming a role model instead of an unfortunate statistic, you can transform the African-American condition into something to which others aspire instead of something that you must endure. Take this information and redefine what it means to be African-American healthy.

Supplement Guidelines

In addition to a comprehensive multivitamin for overall wellness, I recommend the following nutritional supplements to treat the specific illnesses and conditions mentioned throughout this book. Each offers significant benefits and is supported by research.

AGING		
SUPPLEMENT	DOSAGE	CONSIDERATIONS
Alpha-Lipoic Acid	100 to 200 mg three times daily.	If you suffer from thyroid disease, diabetes, or vitamin B_1 deficiency, use alcohol excessively, or are undergoing cancer treatment, talk to your doctor before taking alpha-lipoic acid supplements. Avoid supplementation if you are pregnant or breastfeeding.
Astaxanthin	Follow the manufacturer's instructions.	Avoid supplementation if you are pregnant or breastfeeding.
Blueberry Extract	Follow the manufacturer's instructions.	If you suffer from diabetes, talk to your doctor before taking blueberry extract supplements. Avoid supplementation if you are pregnant or breastfeeding.
Curcumin (BioCurcumin)	250 mg twice daily on an empty stomach.	Avoid supplementation if you are pregnant or breastfeeding, or suffer from gallbladder problems. Stop taking curcumin at least two weeks before any scheduled surgery.
Grape Seed Extract (95 percent OPC)	50 to 200 mg once daily.	Avoid supplementation if you are pregnant or breastfeeding.
N-Acetyl Cysteine (NAC)	600 mg once daily.	If you suffer from asthma, talk to your doctor before taking NAC supplements. Avoid supplementation if you are pregnant or breastfeeding unless absolutely needed. Avoid supplementation if you have an allergy to acetyl cysteine.
Omega-3 Fatty Acids	1,000 mg once daily with food.	If you have problems with your blood pressure, talk to your doctor before taking omega-3 fatty acid supplements.

Pomegranate Extract	250 to 500 mg once daily.	If you are pregnant or breastfeeding, or using any medications, talk to your doctor before taking pomegranate extract. Stop taking pomegranate extract at least two weeks before any scheduled surgery.
Quercitin	500 mg twice daily.	Higher dosages may cause kidney damage. Possible side effects include headaches and tingling of the arms and legs. Avoid supplementation if you are pregnant or breastfeeding.
Resveratrol	20 to 40 mg once daily.	Store supplements in a cool, dry place. Avoid supplementation if you are pregnant or breastfeeding, or suffer from a hormone-sensitive condition, such as breast cancer, uterine cancer, ovarian cancer, endometriosis, or uterine fibroids. Stop taking resveratrol at least two weeks before any scheduled surgery.
Selenium	200 mcg once daily for adults, 60 mcg once daily for women who are pregnant, 70 mcg once daily for women who are breastfeeding.	If you suffer from thyroid disease, have a family history of prostate cancer, or are using proton-pump inhibitors or histamine blockers, talk to your doctor before taking selenium supplements. Possible side effects include reduced fertility in men.
Vitamin C	300 mg once daily for adults, 60 mg once daily for women who are pregnant or breastfeeding.	Higher dosages may cause kidney stones and severe diarrhea. Avoid supplementation if you suffer from sickle cell disease, cancer, hemochromatosis, diabetes, glucose-6-phosphate dehydrogenase (G6PD), or are scheduled for a heart procedure.
Zinc Citrate or Picolinate	15 to 25 mg once daily.	Avoid taking zinc at the same time as calcium, copper, iron, or soy, as it can interfere with the absorption of these nutrients. Zinc supplements can also decrease the absorption of the antibiotics fluoroquinolone and tetracycline.

HYPERTENSION

SUPPLEMENT	DOSAGE	CONSIDERATIONS
Aged Garlic Extract	500 to 600 mg three times daily.	If you are on blood thinners or have a bleeding disorder, talk to your doctor before taking aged garlic extract supplements. Possible side effects include gastrointestinal irritation. Avoid supplementation if you are pregnant or breastfeeding. Stop taking aged garlic extract at least two weeks before any scheduled surgery.

Coenzyme Q$_{10}$ (Ubiquinol)	100 mg one to three times daily with food.	If you have problems with your blood pressure, talk to your doctor before taking coenzyme Q$_{10}$ supplements. Avoid supplementation if you are pregnant or breastfeeding. Stop taking coenzyme Q$_{10}$ at least two weeks before any scheduled surgery.
Dark Chocolate (85 to 99 Percent Cacao)	50 to 100 g daily.	Due to the caffeine content of chocolate, do not eat any more than this amount if you are pregnant or breastfeeding. Possible side effects include anxiety, migraine headaches, increased heart rate, and stomach disturbances. Stop eating dark chocolate at least two weeks before any scheduled surgery.
Grape Seed Extract (95 Percent OPC)	50 to 200 mg once daily.	Avoid supplementation if you are pregnant or breastfeeding.
Hawthorn Berry Extract	160 to 450 mg once or twice daily.	If you are using medications to treat heart disease, talk to your doctor before taking hawthorn berry extract supplements. Avoid supplementation if you are pregnant or breastfeeding.
L-Arginine	1,000 mg once to three times daily.	Possible side effects include diarrhea, nausea, and tightness in the chest. Avoid supplementation if you are pregnant or breastfeeding, suffer from low blood pressure, herpes, asthma, or allergies, or have had a heart attack. Stop taking l-arginine at least two weeks before any scheduled surgery.
L-Carnitine	500 to 1,000 mg twice daily before 3:00 PM.	If you have experienced seizures or suffer from thyroid disease, talk to your doctor before taking l-carnitine supplements.
Lycopene	5 to 20 mg once daily.	Avoid supplementation if you are pregnant or breastfeeding, or have been diagnosed with prostate cancer.
Magnesium Citrate or Glycinate	400 to 800 mg once daily.	Some people experience diarrhea at levels of 600 mg daily and should take less than this amount.
Nattokinase	Follow the manufacturer's instructions.	Avoid supplementation if you are pregnant or breastfeeding, or suffer from a bleeding disorder. Stop taking nattokinase at least two weeks before any scheduled surgery.
Olive Leaf Extract	500 mg twice daily with food.	Avoid supplementation if you are pregnant or breastfeeding.

Omega-3 Fatty Acids	1,000 mg once daily with food.	If you have problems with your blood pressure, talk to your doctor before taking omega-3 fatty acid supplements.
Pomegranate Extract	250 to 500 mg once daily.	If you are pregnant or breastfeeding, or using any medications, talk to your doctor before taking pomegranate extract. Stop taking pomegranate extract at least two weeks before any scheduled surgery.
Vitamin D₃	2,000 to 5,000 IU once daily.	Talk to your doctor before taking vitamin D_3 supplements at levels above 1,000 IU daily.
Vitamin E (Mixed Tocopherols & Tocotrienols)	100 to 400 IU once daily.	If you are using blood thinners, talk to your doctor before taking vitamin E supplements.
Vitamin K₂	70 to 80 mcg once daily for men, 55 to 65 mcg once daily for women.	If you suffer from kidney or liver disease, talk to your doctor before taking vitamin K_2 supplements.

CANCER

SUPPLEMENT	DOSAGE	CONSIDERATIONS
Alpha-Lipoic Acid	100 to 200 mg three times daily.	If you suffer from thyroid disease, diabetes, or vitamin B_1 deficiency, use alcohol excessively, or are undergoing cancer treatment, talk to your doctor before taking alpha-lipoic acid supplements. Avoid supplementation if you are pregnant or breastfeeding.
Andrographis	400 mg twice daily for no more than fourteen days at a time.	If you are undergoing cancer treatment, talk to your doctor before taking andrographis supplements. Avoid supplementation if you are pregnant or breastfeeding, have fertility problems, or suffer from an autoimmune disease, such as multiple sclerosis, lupus, or rheumatoid arthritis.
Astaxanthin	Follow the manufacturer's instructions.	Avoid supplementation if you are pregnant or breastfeeding.
Black Raspberry Extract	Follow the manufacturer's instructions.	Avoid supplementation if you are pregnant or breastfeeding.
Blueberry Extract	Follow the manufacturer's instructions.	If you suffer from diabetes, talk to your doctor before taking blueberry extract supplements. Avoid supplementation if you are pregnant or breastfeeding.
Curcumin (BioCurcumin)	250 mg twice daily on an empty stomach.	Avoid supplementation if you are pregnant or breastfeeding, or have gallbladder problems. Stop taking curcumin at least two weeks before any scheduled surgery.

Echinacea	250 to 500 mg for no more than eight weeks at a time.	If you are undergoing cancer treatment, talk to your doctor before taking echinacea supplements. Possible side effects include dizziness and nausea. Avoid supplementation if you are pregnant or breastfeeding, have a tendency towards allergies, or suffer from an autoimmune disease, such as multiple sclerosis, lupus, rheumatoid arthritis, or pemphigus vulgaris.
Elderberry Extract	Follow the manufacturer's instructions.	Avoid supplementation if you are pregnant or breastfeeding, or suffer from an autoimmune disease, such as multiple sclerosis, lupus, or rheumatoid arthritis.
Grape Seed Extract (95 percent OPC)	50 to 200 mg once daily.	Avoid supplementation if you are pregnant or breastfeeding.
Green Tea Extract	6 to 9 drops added to 32 ounces of water to be ingested throughout the day.	If you suffer from diabetes, osteoporosis, or glaucoma, talk to your doctor before taking green tea extract. Avoid supplementation if you suffer from a bleeding disorder, anxiety disorder, anemia, heart problems, or liver disease.
N-Acetyl Cysteine (NAC)	600 mg once daily.	If you suffer from asthma, talk to your doctor before taking NAC supplements. Avoid supplementation if you are pregnant or breastfeeding unless absolutely needed. Avoid supplementation if you have an allergy to acetyl cysteine.
Olive Leaf Extract	500 mg twice daily with food.	Avoid supplementation if you are pregnant or breastfeeding.
Pomegranate Extract	250 to 500 mg once daily.	If you are pregnant or breastfeeding, or using any medications, talk to your doctor before taking pomegranate extract. Stop taking pomegranate extract at least two weeks before any scheduled surgery.
Quercitin	500 mg twice daily.	Higher dosages may cause kidney damage. Possible side effects include headaches and tingling of the arms and legs. Avoid supplementation if you are pregnant or breastfeeding.
Resveratrol	20 to 40 mg once daily.	Store supplements in a cool, dry place. Avoid supplementation if you are pregnant or breastfeeding, or suffer from a hormone-sensitive condition, such as breast cancer, uterine cancer, ovarian cancer, endometriosis, or uterine fibroids. Stop taking resveratrol at least two weeks before any scheduled surgery.

Selenium	200 mcg once daily for adults, 60 mcg once daily for women who are pregnant, 70 mcg once daily for women who are breastfeeding.	If you suffer from thyroid disease, have a family history of prostate cancer, or are using proton-pump inhibitors or histamine blockers, talk to your doctor before taking selenium supplements. Possible side effects include reduced fertility in men.
Vitamin C	300 mg once daily for adults, 60 mg once daily for women who are pregnant or breastfeeding.	Higher dosages may cause kidney stones and severe diarrhea. Avoid supplementation if you suffer from sickle cell disease, cancer, hemo-chromatosis, diabetes, or glucose-6-phosphate dehydrogenase (G6PD), or are scheduled for a heart procedure.
Vitamin D_3	2,000 to 5,000 IU once daily.	Talk to your doctor before taking vitamin D_3 supplements at levels above 1,000 IU daily.
Zinc Citrate or Picolinate	15 to 25 mg once daily.	Avoid taking zinc at the same time as calcium, copper, iron, or soy, as it can interfere with the absorption of these nutrients. Zinc supplements can also decrease the absorption of the antibiotics fluoroquinolone and tetracycline.

STROKE

SUPPLEMENT	DOSAGE	CONSIDERATIONS
Aged Garlic Extract	500 to 600 mg three times daily.	If you are on blood thinners or have a bleeding disorder, talk to your doctor before taking aged garlic extract supplements. Possible side effects include gastrointestinal irritation. Avoid supplementation if you are pregnant or breastfeeding. Stop taking aged garlic extract at least two weeks before any scheduled surgery.
Coenzyme Q_{10} (Ubiquinol)	100 mg once to three times daily with food.	If you have problems with your blood pressure, talk to your doctor before taking coenzyme Q_{10} supplements. Avoid supplementation if you are pregnant or breastfeeding. Stop taking coenzyme Q_{10} at least two weeks before any scheduled surgery.
Dark Chocolate (85 to 99 Percent Cacao)	50 to 100 g daily.	Due to the caffeine content of chocolate, do not eat any more than this amount if you are pregnant or breastfeeding. Possible side effects include anxiety, migraine headaches, increased heart rate, and stomach disturbances. Stop eating dark chocolate at least two weeks before any scheduled surgery.

Grape Seed Extract (95 percent OPC)	50 to 200 mg once daily.	Avoid supplementation if you are pregnant or breastfeeding.
Hawthorn Berry Extract	160 to 450 mg once or twice daily.	If you are using medications to treat heart disease, talk to your doctor before taking hawthorn berry extract supplements. Avoid supplementation if you are pregnant or breastfeeding.
L-Arginine	1,000 mg once to three times daily.	Possible side effects include diarrhea, nausea, and tightness in the chest. Avoid supplementation if you are pregnant or breastfeeding, suffer from low blood pressure, herpes, asthma, or allergies, or have had a heart attack. Stop taking l-arginine at least two weeks before any scheduled surgery.
L-Carnitine	500 to 1,000 mg twice daily before 3:00 PM.	If you have experienced seizures or suffer from thyroid disease, talk to your doctor before taking l-carnitine supplements.
Lycopene	5 to 20 mg once daily.	Avoid supplementation if you are pregnant or breastfeeding, or have been diagnosed with prostate cancer.
Magnesium Citrate or Glycinate	400 to 800 mg once daily.	Some people experience diarrhea at levels of 600 mg daily and should take less than this amount.
Nattokinase	Follow the manufacturer's instructions.	Avoid supplementation if you are pregnant or breastfeeding, or suffer from a bleeding disorder. Stop taking nattokinase at least two weeks before any scheduled surgery.
Omega-3 Fatty Acids	1,000 mg once daily with food.	If you have problems with your blood pressure, talk to your doctor before taking omega-3 fatty acid supplements.
Pomegranate Extract	250 to 500 mg once daily.	If you are pregnant or breastfeeding, or using any medications, talk to your doctor before taking pomegranate extract. Stop taking pomegranate extract at least two weeks before any scheduled surgery.
Vitamin B Complex	15 mg of B_3, 2 mg of B_6, 400 mcg of B_9, and 2.4 mcg of B_{12} once daily.	If you have low blood pressure, stomach ulcers, or diabetes, or suffer from kidney, liver, gallbladder, or heart disease, talk to your doctor before taking vitamin B_3 supplements. Avoid supplementation with vitamin B_{12} if you are allergic to cobalt or cobalamin, or suffer from Leber's disease.
Vitamin D_3	2,000 to 5,000 IU once daily.	Talk to your doctor before taking vitamin D_3 supplements at levels above 1,000 IU daily.

TYPE 2 DIABETES

SUPPLEMENT	DOSAGE	CONSIDERATIONS
Alpha-Lipoic Acid	100 to 200 mg three times daily.	If you suffer from thyroid disease, diabetes, or vitamin B_1 deficiency, use alcohol excessively, or are undergoing cancer treatment, talk to your doctor before taking alpha-lipoic acid supplements. Avoid supplementation if you are pregnant or breastfeeding.
Chromium Picolinate	50 to 200 mcg once daily.	Higher dosages to treat specific diseases should be discussed with your doctor. Avoid supplementation if you suffer from diabetes, liver or kidney disease, behavioral or psychiatric conditions, or chromate or leather allergies, or are pregnant or breastfeeding.
Cinnulin PF	125 to 150 mg three times daily.	If you suffer from diabetes, talk to your doctor before taking Cinnulin PF supplements. Avoid supplementation if you are pregnant or breastfeeding, or suffer from liver disease. Stop taking Cinnulin PF at least two weeks before any scheduled surgery.
Coenzyme Q_{10} (Ubiquinol)	100 mg once to three times daily with food.	If you have problems with your blood pressure, talk to your doctor before taking coenzyme Q_{10} supplements. Avoid supplementation if you are pregnant or breastfeeding. Stop taking coenzyme Q_{10} at least two weeks before any scheduled surgery.
DHEA	50 to 100 mg once daily for men, 25 mg once daily for women. Get your DHEA level checked by your doctor for a personalized dosage.	Avoid supplementation if you are pregnant or breastfeeding, or suffer from liver problems, polycystic ovary syndrome, or a hormone-sensitive condition, such as breast cancer, uterine cancer, ovarian cancer, endometriosis, uterine fibroids, or prostate cancer. If you suffer from diabetes, mood disorder, or cholesterol problems, talk to your doctor before taking DHEA supplements.
Green Tea Extract	6 to 9 drops added to 32 ounces of water to be ingested throughout the day.	If you suffer from diabetes, osteoporosis, or glaucoma, talk to your doctor before taking green tea extract supplements. Avoid supplementation if you suffer from a bleeding disorder, anxiety disorder, anemia, heart problems, or liver disease.

Gymnema Silvestre	Follow the manufacturer's instructions.	If you suffer from diabetes, talk to your doctor before taking gymnema silvestre supplements. Avoid supplementation if you are pregnant or breastfeeding. Stop taking gymnema silvestre at least two weeks before any scheduled surgery.
L-Carnitine	500 to 1,000 mg twice daily before 3:00 PM.	If you have experienced seizures or suffer from thyroid disease, talk to your doctor before taking l-carnitine supplements.
Vitamin D_3	2,000 to 5,000 IU once daily.	Talk to your doctor before taking vitamin D_3 supplements at levels above 1,000 IU daily.

KIDNEY DISEASE

SUPPLEMENT	DOSAGE	CONSIDERATIONS
DHEA	50 to 100 mg once daily for men, 25 mg once daily for women. Get your DHEA level checked by your doctor for a personalized dosage.	Avoid supplementation if you are pregnant or breastfeeding, or suffer from liver problems, polycystic ovary syndrome, or a hormone-sensitive condition, such as breast cancer, uterine cancer, ovarian cancer, endometriosis, uterine fibroids, or prostate cancer. If you suffer from diabetes, mood disorder, or cholesterol problems, talk to your doctor before taking DHEA supplements.
L-Theanine	50 to 200 mg once daily.	Avoid supplementation if you are pregnant or breastfeeding.
Vitamin D_3	2,000 to 5,000 IU once daily.	Talk to your doctor before taking vitamin D_3 supplements at levels above 1,000 IU daily.
Vitamin K_2	70 to 80 mcg once daily for men, 55 to 65 mcg once daily for women.	If you suffer from kidney or liver disease, talk to your doctor before taking vitamin K_2 supplements.

OBESITY

SUPPLEMENT	DOSAGE	CONSIDERATIONS
5-Hydroxy-tryptophan (5-HTP)	50 mg twice to three times daily.	Possible side effects include heartburn, stomach ache, nausea, vomiting, diarrhea, drowsiness, muscular problems, and sexual problems. Avoid supplementation if you are pregnant or breastfeeding, or have Down syndrome.
Coenzyme Q_{10} (Ubiquinol)	100 mg once to three times daily with food.	If you have problems with your blood pressure, talk to your doctor before taking coenzyme Q_{10} supplements. Avoid supplementation if you are pregnant or breastfeeding. Stop taking coenzyme Q_{10} at least two weeks before any scheduled surgery.

Glisodin	150 mg once or twice daily.	Talk to your doctor before taking glisodin supplements.
Green Tea Extract	6 to 9 drops added to 32 ounces of water to be ingested throughout the day.	If you suffer from diabetes, osteoporosis, or glaucoma, talk to your doctor before taking green tea extract supplements. Avoid supplementation if you suffer from a bleeding disorder, anxiety disorder, anemia, heart problems, or liver disease.
Greens Powder	Follow the manufacturer's instructions.	Talk to your doctor before taking greens powder supplements.
Irvingia Gabonensis	150 mg twice daily.	Possible side effects include flatulence, headaches, and sleep problems. Avoid supplementation if you are pregnant or breastfeeding.
L-Carnitine	500 to 1,000 mg twice daily before 3:00 PM.	If you have experienced seizures or suffer from thyroid disease, talk to your doctor before taking l-carnitine supplements.
L-Theanine	50 to 200 mg once daily.	Avoid supplementation if you are pregnant or breastfeeding.
Reds Powder	Follow the manufacturer's instructions.	Talk to your doctor before taking reds powder supplements.
Saffron	30 mg twice daily.	Possible side effects include dry mouth, anxiety, dizziness, nausea, fatigue, headaches, and a change in appetite. Avoid supplementation if you are pregnant or breastfeeding, suffer from a bipolar disorder, or are allergic to the plant species Lolia, Olea, or Salsola.

MEN'S HEALTH

SUPPLEMENT	DOSAGE	CONSIDERATIONS
Beta-Sitosterol	20 to 40 mg three times daily.	Avoid supplementation if you suffer from sitosterolomia.
Diindolylmethane (DIM)	Follow the manufacturer's instructions.	Avoid supplementation if you suffer from a hormone-sensitive condition, such as prostate cancer.
Flax Lignans	10 to 30 mg once daily.	If you suffer from diabetes, gastrointestinal obstruction, or a hormone-sensitive condition, such as prostate cancer, talk to your doctor before taking flax lignans. Avoid supplementation if you have high triglycerides or suffer from a bleeding disorder.
Green Tea Extract	6 to 9 drops added to 32 ounces of water to be ingested throughout the day.	If you suffer from diabetes, osteoporosis, or glaucoma, talk to your doctor before taking green tea extract. Avoid supplementation if you suffer from a bleeding disorder, anxiety disorder, anemia, heart problems, or liver disease.

HMRlignans	10 to 30 mg once daily.	If you suffer from diabetes, gastrointestinal obstruction, or a hormone-sensitive condition, such as prostate cancer, talk to your doctor before taking HMRlignans. Avoid supplementation if you have high triglycerides or suffer from a bleeding disorder.
Indole-3-Carbinol	200 to 400 mg once daily.	Higher dosages may cause balance problems, tremors, and nausea.
Lycopene	5 to 20 mg once daily.	Avoid supplementation if you have been diagnosed with prostate cancer.
Saw Palmetto	160 mg twice daily.	Possible side effects include dizziness, headaches, nausea, vomiting, constipation, and diarrhea. Stop taking saw palmetto at least two weeks before any scheduled surgery.
Selenium	200 mcg once daily.	If you suffer from thyroid disease, have a family history of prostate cancer, or are using proton-pump inhibitors or histamine blockers, talk to your doctor before taking selenium supplements. Possible side effects include reduced fertility in men.
Vitamin D_3	2,000 to 5,000 IU once daily.	Talk to your doctor before taking vitamin D_3 supplements at levels above 1,000 IU daily.
Zinc Citrate or Picolinate	15 to 25 mg once daily.	Avoid taking zinc at the same time as calcium, copper, iron, or soy, as it can interfere with the absorption of these nutrients. Zinc supplements can also decrease the absorption of the antibiotics fluoroquinolone and tetracycline.

WOMEN'S HEALTH

SUPPLEMENT	DOSAGE	CONSIDERATIONS
Calcium	Daily calcium intake should be about 1,000 mg per day from both diet and supplementation.	Calcium supplements can decrease the absorption of aluminum, magnesium, zinc, iron, manganese, phosphorus, thyroid medication, and the antibiotics ciprofloxacin, fluoroquinolone, and tetracycline. Talk to your doctor before starting supplementation.
Diindolyl-methane (DIM)	Follow the manufacturer's instructions.	Avoid supplementation if you are pregnant or breastfeeding, or suffer from a hormone-sensitive condition, such as breast cancer, uterine cancer, ovarian cancer, endometriosis, or uterine fibroids.

Flax Lignans	10 to 30 mg once daily.	If you suffer from diabetes, gastrointestinal obstruction, or a hormone-sensitive condition, such as breast cancer, uterine cancer, ovarian cancer, endometriosis, or uterine fibroids, talk to your doctor before taking flax lignans. Avoid supplementation if you are pregnant or breastfeeding, have high triglycerides, or suffer from a bleeding disorder.
Green Tea Extract	6 to 9 drops added to 32 ounces of water to be ingested throughout the day.	If you suffer from diabetes, osteoporosis, or glaucoma, talk to your doctor before taking green tea extract. Avoid supplementation if you suffer from a bleeding disorder, anxiety disorder, anemia, heart problems, or liver disease.
HMRlignans	10 to 30 mg once daily.	If you suffer from diabetes, gastrointestinal obstruction, or a hormone-sensitive condition, such as breast cancer, uterine cancer, ovarian cancer, endometriosis, or uterine fibroids, talk to your doctor before taking HMRlignans. Avoid supplementation if you are pregnant or breastfeeding, have high triglycerides, or suffer from a bleeding disorder.
Indole-3-Carbinol	200 to 400 mg once daily.	Higher dosages may cause balance problems, tremors, and nausea. Avoid supplementation if you are pregnant or breastfeeding.
Lycopene	5 to 20 mg once daily.	Avoid supplementation if you are pregnant or breastfeeding.
Vitamin D_3	2,000 to 5,000 IU once daily.	Talk to your doctor before taking vitamin D_3 supplements at levels above 1,000 IU daily.

References

Chapter 1

1. www.minorityhealth.hhs.gov

2. www.americanheart.org

3. www.med.nyu.edu

4. www.blackhealthcare.com

5. "Health Care Spending in the United States and OECD Countries." www.kff.org

6. Gamble, V. N. "Under the shadow of Tuskegee: African Americans and health care." *American Journal of Public Health* (1997): Vol. 87, no. 11, 1773–1778.

7. Rajakumar, K, et al. "Racial Differences in Parents' Distrust of Medicine and Research." *Archives of Pediatrics & Adolescent Medicine* (2009): Vol. 163, no. 2, 108–114.

8. Thomas, S. B. and Quinn, S. C. "The AIDS Epidemic and the African-American Community: Toward an Ethical Framework for Service Delivery." In *"It Just Ain't Fair"*: *The Ethics of Health Care for African Americans,* edited by A. Dula and S. Goering. New York: Praeger, 1994.

9. Richardson, L. "An Old Experiment's Legacy: Distrust of AIDS Treatment." *The New York Times,* 21 April 1997, Al, A7.

10. "Vitamin D deficiency soars in the U.S., study says." www.scientificamerican.com

Chapter 2

1. "Vitamin D Protects Cells from Stress." *The International Journal of Cancer* (2009): Vol. 124, no. 12.

2. *American Society of Clinical Oncology's Breast Cancer Symposium,* 2009.

Chapter 3

1. Bender, D. A. *Nutritional Biochemistry of the Vitamins.* Cambridge, UK: Cambridge University Press, 2003.

2. Bolander, F. F. "Vitamins: not just for enzymes." *Curr Opin Investig Drugs* (2006): Vol. 7, no. 10, 912–915.

3. *The Kirk-Othmer Encyclopedia of Chemical Technology Third Edition.* New York: John Wiley and Sons, 1984: Vol. 24, 104.

4. Norman, A. W. "Sunlight, season, skin pigmentation, vitamin D, and 25-hydroxyvitamin D: integral components of the vitamin D endocrine system." *Am J Clin Nutr* (1998): Vol. 67, no. 6, 1108–1110.

5. Putnis, A. *Introduction to Mineral Sciences.* Cambridge, UK: Cambridge University Press, 1992.

6. Guryev, O, et al. "A pathway for the metabolism of vitamin D3: "Unique hydroxylated metabolites formed during catalysis with cytochrome P450scc (CYP11A1)." *PNAS* (2003): Vol. 100, no. 25, 14754–14759.

7. Lappe, J, et al. "Vitamin D and calcium supplementation reduces cancer risk: results of a randomized trial" *Am J Clin Nutr* (2007): Vol. 85, no. 6, 1586–1591.

8. Hoogendijk, Witte J. G. "Depression Is Associated With Decreased 25-Hydroxyvitamin D and Increased Parathyroid Hormone Levels in Older Adults." *American Medical Association Journal Archives of General Psychiatry* (2008): Vol. 65, no. 5.

9. von Hurst, P. R. "Vitamin D supplementation reduces insulin resistance in South Asian women living in New Zealand who are insulin resistant and vitamin D deficient - a randomised, placebo-controlled trial." *Br J Nutr* (2010): Vol. 103, no. 4, 549–555.

10. "Study Finds Low Vitamin D in Children." www.news.aol.com

11. Scragg, R, et al. "Serum 25-hydroxyvitamin D, ethnicity, and blood pressure in the Third National Health and Nutrition Examination Survey." *American Journal of Hypertension* (2007): Vol. 20, no. 7, 713–719.

12. Giovannucci, E, et al. "25-Hydroxyvitamin D and Risk of Myocardial Infarction in Men. A Prospective Study." *Arch Intern Med* (2008): Vol. 168, no. 11,1174–1180.

13. *American Medical Association Journal Archives of General Psychiatry* (2008): Vol. 65, no. 5.

Chapter 4

1. *Cecil Textbook of Medicine 22nd Edition.* Philadelphia: Saunders, 2004.

2. *Lancet* (1990): Vol. 335, 1092–1094.

3. Li, Y. C, et al. "Vitamin D: a negative endocrine regulator of the renin–angiotensin system and blood pressure." References and further reading may be available for this article. To view references and further reading you must purchase this article. *J Steroid Biochem Mol Biol* (2004): Vol. 89–90, no. 1–5, 387-392.

4. Scragg, R, et al. "Serum 25-hydroxyvitamin D, ethnicity, and blood pressure in the Third National Health and Nutrition Examination Survey." *American Journal of Hypertension* (2007): Vol. 20, no. 7, 713–719.

5. Ford, E. S. "Does exercise reduce inflammation? Physical activity and C-reactive protein among U.S. adults." *Epidemiology* (2002): Vol. 13, no. 5, 561–568.

6. Franklin, B, et al. "Effects of a contemporary, exercise-based rehabilitation and cardiovascular risk-reduction program on coronary patients with abnormal baseline risk factors." *Chest* (2002): Vol. 122, no. 1, 338–343.

7. Carroll, S. and Dudfield, M. "What is the Relationship Between Exercise and Metabolic Abnormalities?: A Review of the Metabolic Syndrome." *Sports Medicine* (2004): Vol. 34, no. 6, 371–418.

8. von Kanel, R, et al. "Effects of psychological stress and psychiatric disorders on blood coagulation and fibrinolysis: a biobehavioral pathway to coronary artery disease?" *Psychosom Med* (2001): Vol. 63, no. 4, 531–544.

9. "'John Henryism' Key to Understanding Coping, Health." www.duke health.org

Chapter 5

1. Morgan, C, et al. "Detection of p53 mutations in precancerous gastric tissue." *British Journal of Cancer* (2003): Vol. 89, 1314–1319.

2. Wood, K. A. and Youle, R. J. "The role of free radicals and p53 in neuron apoptosis in vivo." *Journal of Neuroscience* (1995): Vol. 15, 5851–5857.

3. Pogribny, I. P, et al. "Breaks in Genomic DNA and within the p53 Gene Are Associated with Hypomethylation in Livers of Folate/methyl-deficient Rats." *Cancer Research* (1995): Vol. 55, 1894–1901.

4. John E, et al. "Vitamin D and breast cancer risk: The NHANES I epidemiologic follow-up study, 1971–1975 to 1992." *Cancer Epidemiol Biomarkers Prev* (1999): Vol. 8, 399–406.

5. Freedman, D. M, et al. "Prospective study of serum vitamin D and cancer mortality in the United States." *J Natl Cancer Inst* (2007): Vol. 99, 1594–1602.

6. www.cancer.org

7. Albertsen, P. C. "20-Year outcomes following conservative management of clinically localized prostate cancer" *JAMA* (2005): Vol. 293, no.17, 2095–2101.

8. Li, H, et al. "A Prospective Study of Plasma Vitamin D Metabolites, Vitamin D Receptor Polymorphisms, and Prostate Cancer." *PLoS Medicine* (2007): Vol. 4, no. 3, 103.

9. Dawson-Hughes, B, et al. "Estimates of optimal vitamin D status." *Osteoporosis International* (2005): Vol. 16, 713–717.

10. Garland, C. F, et al. "What is the dose response relationship between vitamin D and cancer risk?" *Nutrition Reviews* (2007):Vol. 65, no. 8, S91–S95.

11. Freedman, D. M, et al. "Prospective study of serum vitamin D and cancer mortality in the United States." *J Natl Cancer Inst* (2007): Vol. 99, 1594–1602.

12. Gorham, E. D, et al. "Optimal vitamin D status for colorectal cancer prevention: a quantitative meta analysis." *Am J Prev Med* (2007): Vol. 32, 210–216.

13. Lefkowitz, E. S. and Garland C. F. "Sunlight, vitamin D, and ovarian cancer mortality rates in US women." *Int J Epidemiol* (1994): Vol. 23, 1133–1136.

14. Grant, W. B. "Ecologic studies of solar UV-B radiation and cancer mortality rates." *Recent Results Cancer Res* (2003): Vol. 164, 371–377.

15. Garland, C, et al. "Role of ultraviolet B irradiance and vitamin D in prevention of ovarian cancer." *Am J Prev Med* (2006): Vol. 31, 512–514.

16. Garland, C. F. "Vitamin D for cancer prevention" *AEP* (2009): Vol. 19, no. 7, 468–483.

17. Grant, W. B. and Garland, C. F. "The association of solar ultraviolet B (UVB) with reducing risk of cancer: multifactorial ecologic analysis of geographic variation in age-adjusted cancer mortality rates." *Anticancer Res* (2006): Vol. 26, 2687–2699.

Chapter 6

1. "Strokes will cost U.S. $2.2 trillion over the next 45 years." www.neuro logy.org

2. Zivin, J. A. "Approaches to Cerebrovascular Disease." In *Cecil Textbook of Medicine 22nd ed.*, edited by Goldman and Ausiello. Philadelphia: Saunders Elsevier, 2007.

3. Ross, R. "Atherosclerosis – An inflammatory Disease." *NEJM* (1999): Vol. 340, 115–126.

4. Pasceri, V, et al. "Direct Proinflammatory Effect of C-Reactive Protein on Human Endothelial Cells." *Circulation* (2000): Vol. 102, 2165–2168.

5. Mulvihill, N. T. and Foley, J. B. "Inflammation in acute coronary syndromes." *Heart* (2002): Vol. 87,201–204.

6. Ford, E. S. "Does exercise reduce inflammation? Physical activity and the C-Reactive protein among U.S. adults." *Epidemiology* (2002). Vol. 13, no. 5, 561–568.

7. Zhu, J, et al. "Prospective Study of Pathogen Burden and Risk of Myocardial Infarction or Death. Clinical Investigation and Reports." *Circulation* (2001): Vol.103, no. 1, 45–51.

8. George, J. "The Prediction of coronary atherosclerosis employing artificial neural networks." *Clinical Cardiology* (2000): Vol. 23, no. 6, 453–456.

9. Muntner, P, et al. "Blood lead and chronic kidney disease in the general United States population: results from NHANES III." *Kidney Int* (2003): Vol. 63, 1044–1050.

10. Rissanen, T, et al. "Fish Oil–Derived Fatty Acids, Docosahexaenoic Acid and Docosapentaenoic Acid, and the Risk of Acute Coronary Events: The Kuopio Ischaemic Heart Disease Risk Factor Study." *Circulation* (2000): Vol. 102, no. 22, 2677–2679.

11. Sorensen, N. "Prenatal methylmercury exposure as a cardiovascular risk factor at seven years of age." *Epidemiology* (1999): Vol. 10, no. 4, 370–375.

12. Salonene, J. T, et al. "Intake of Mercury From Fish, Lipid Peroxidation, and the Risk of Myocardial Infarction and Coronary, Cardiovascular, and Any Death in Eastern Finnish Men." *Circulation* (1995): Vol. 91, no. 3, 645–655.

13. Köster, R, et al. Nickel and molybdenum contact allergies in patients with coronary in-stent restenosis." *Lancet* (2000): Vol. 356, no. 9245, 1895–1897.

14. "African Americans and Stroke." www.stroke.org

15. Pilz, S, et al. "Low vitamin d levels predict stroke in patients referred to coronary angiography." *Stroke* (2008): Vol. 39, no. 9, 2611–2613.

16. Poole, K. E, et al. "Reduced vitamin D in acute stroke." *Stroke* (2006): Vol. 37, no. 1, 243–245.

17. McIlroy, S. P, et al. "Moderately Elevated Plasma Homocysteine, Methylenetetrahydrofolate Reductase Genotype, and Risk for Stroke, Vascular Dementia, and Alzheimer Disease in Northern Ireland." *Stroke* (2002): Vol. 33, 2351.

18. Wynn, M. and Wynn, A. "Fortification of grain products with folate: should Britain follow the American example." *Nutr Health* (1998): Vol. 12, no. 3, 147–161.

19. Yang, Q. "Improvement in stroke mortality in Canada and the United States, 1990 to 2002." *Circulation* (2006): Vol. 113, no. 10, 1335–1343.

Chapter 7

1. Laditka S. B, et al. "Health care use of individuals with diabetes in an employer-based insurance population." *Arch Intern Med* (2001): Vol. 161, no. 10, 1301–1308.

2. "Diabetes Mellitus, Type 2 - A Review." www.emedicine.com

3. Wright, E, et al. "Oxidative stress in type 2 diabetes: the role of fasting and postprandial gylcemia." *Int J Clin Pract* (2006): Vol. 60, no. 3, 308–314.

4. "Diabetes Mellitus, Type 2 - A Review." www.emedicine.com

5. Littorin, B, et al. "Lower levels of plasma 25-hydroxyvitamin D among young adults at diagnosis of autoimmune type 1 diabetes compared with control subjects: results from the nationwide Diabetes Incidence Study in Sweden (DISS)." *Diabetologia* (2006): Vol. 49, no. 12, 2847–2852.

6. Duncan, B, et al. "Low-Grade Systemic Inflammation and the Development of Type 2 Diabetes: The Atherosclerosis Risk in Communities Study." *Diabetes* (2003): Vol. 52, no. 7, 1799–1805.

7. Csiszar, A, and Ungvari, Z. "Endothelial dysfunction and vascular inflammation in Type 2 diabetes: interaction of AGE/RAGE and TNF- signaling." *Am J Physiol Heart Circ Physiol* (2008): Vol. 295, no. 2, H475–H476.

8. Filus, A, et al. "Relationship between vitamin D receptor BsmI and FokI polymorphisms and anthropometric and biochemical parameters describing metabolic syndrome." *Aging Male* (2008): Vol. 11, no. 3, 134–139.

9. Lee, J. H, et al. "Vitamin D deficiency an important, common, and easily treatable cardiovascular risk factor?" *J Am Coll Cardiol* (2008): Vol. 52, no. 24, 1949–1956.

10. Alemzadeh, R, et al. "Hypovitaminosis D in obese children and adolescents:

relationship with adiposity, insulin sensitivity, ethnicity, and season." *Metabolism* (2008): Vol. 57, no. 2, 183–191.

11. Penckofer, S, et al. "Vitamin D and diabetes: let the sunshine in." *Diabetes Educ* (2008): Vol. 34, no. 6, 939–944.

12. Zittermann, A, et al. "Circulating calcitriol concentrations and total mortality." *Clin Chem* (2009): Vol. 55, no. 6, 1163–1170.

13. Wright, E, et al. "Oxidative stress in type 2 diabetes: the role of fasting and postprandial gylcemia." *Int J Clin Pract* (2006): Vol. 60, no. 3, 308–314.

14. Alfonso, B, et al. "Vitamin D in diabetes mellitus-a new field of knowledge poised for D-velopment." *Diabetes Metab Res Rev* (2009): Vol. 25, no. 5, 417–419.

15. Mingrone, G. "Carnitine in Type 2 Diabetes." *Annals of the New York Academy of Sciences* (2004): Vol. 1033, 99–107.

16. Guideri, F, et al. "Effects of Acetyl-L-carnitine on Cardiac Dysautonomia in Rett Syndrome: Prevention of Sudden Death?" *Pediatric Cardiology* (2005): Vol. 26, no. 5, 574–577.

17. Ghosh, D, et al. "Role of chromium supplementation in Indians with type 2 diabetes mellitus." *The Journal of Nutritional Biochemistry* (2002): Vol. 13, no. 11, 690–697.

18. Anderson, R. A, and Preuss, H. G. "Chromium update: examining recent literature 1997–1998." *Current Opinion in Clinical Nutrition and Metabolic Care* (1998): Vol. 1, no. 6, 509–512.

19. Anderson, R. A, et al. "Isolation and Characterization of Polyphenol Type-A Polymers from Cinnamon with Insulin-like Biological Activity." *J Agri Food Chem* (2004): Vol. 52, no. 1, 65–70.

20. Imparl-Radosevich, J, et al. "Regulation of PTP-1 and insulin receptor kinase by fractions from cinnamon: implications for cinnamon regulation of insulin signaling." *Horm Res* (1998): Vol. 50, no. 3, 177–182.

21. Hodgson, J. M. and Watts, G. F. "Can coenzyme Q10 improve vascular function and blood pressure? Potential for effective therapeutic reduction in vascular oxidative stress." *BioFactors* (2003): Vol. 18, no. 1–4/2003, 129–136.

22. Watts, G. F, et al. "Coenzyme Q10 improves endothelial dysfunction of the brachial artery in Type II diabetes mellitus." *Diabetologia* (2002): Vol. 45, no. 3, 420–426.

23. Al-Thakafy, H. S, et al. "Alterations of erythrocyte free radical defense system, heart tissue lipid peroxidation, and lipid concentration in streptozotocin-induced diabetic rats under coenzyme Q10 supplementation." *Saudi Med J* (2004): Vol. 25, no. 12, 1824–1830.

24. Yamashita, R, et al. "Effects of dehydroepiandrosterone on gluconeogenic enzymes and glucose uptake in human hepatoma cell line, HepG2." *Endocr J* (2005): Vol. 52, no. 6, 727–753.

25. Boudou, P, et al. "Hyperglycaemia acutely decreases circulating dehydroepiandrosterone levels in healthy men." *Clinical Endocrinology* (2006): Vol. 64, no. 1, 46–52.

26. Jones, R. D, et al. "Testosterone and Atherosclerosis in Aging Men: Purported Association and Clinical Implications." *American Journal of Cardiovascular Drugs* (2005): Vol. 56, no. 3, 141–154.

27. Medina M. C, et al. "Dehydroepiandrosterone increases beta-cell mass and improves the glucose-induced insulin secretion by pancreatic islets from aged rats." *FEBS Lett* (2006): Vol. 580, no. 1, 285–290.

28. Chandalia, M, et al. "Beneficial effects of high dietary fiber intake in patients with type 2 diabetes mellitus." *New England Journal of Medicine* (2000): Vol. 342, 1392–1398.

29. Okuda, T, et al. "Inhibitory effect of tannins on direct-acting mutation." *Chem Pharm Bull* (1984): Vol. 32, 3755–3758.

30. Crespy, V. and Williamson, G. A. "Review of the health effects of green tea catechins in in vivo animal models." *J Nutr* (2004): Vol. 134, 3431S–3440S.

31. Nurulain, T. Z. "Green tea and its polyphenolic catechins: Medicinal uses in cancer and noncancer applications." *Life Sciences* (2006): Vol. 78, no. 18, 2073–2080.

32. "Drug Interaction Checker." www.drugs.com

33. Murase, T, et al. "Green tea extract improves endurance capacity and increases muscle lipid oxidation in mice." *Am J Physiol Regul Integr Comp Physiol* (2005): Vol. 288, R708–R715.

34. Henriksen, E. J, et al. "Stimulation by alpha-lipoic acid of glucose transport activity in skeletal muscle of lean and obese zucker rats." *Life Sciences* (1997): Vol. 61, no. 8, 805–812.

35. www.healthy4youonline.com

Chapter 8

1. Norris, K. C. and Francis, C. K. "Gender and ethnic differences and considerations in cardiovascular risk assessment and prevention in African Americans." *Practical Strategies in Preventing Heart Disease*. New York: McGraw-Hill, 2000.

2. Martins, D. and Norris, K. "Hypertension treatment in African Americans: Physiology is less important than sociology." *Cleveland Clinical J of Medicine* (2004): Vol. 71, no. 9, 735-743.

3. Freedman, B, et al. "Familial predisposition to nephropathy in African-Americans with non-insulin-dependent diabetes mellitus." *American Journal of Kidney Diseases* (1995): Vol. 25, no. 5, 710–713.

4. Bergman, S, et al. "Kidney disease in the first-degree relatives of African-Americans with hypertensive end-stage renal disease." *American Journal of Kidney Diseases* (1996): Vol. 27, no. 3, 341–346.

5. Suthanthiran, M, et al. "Transforming growth factor-beta hyperexpression in African-American hypertensives: A novel mediator of hypertension and/or target organ damage." *PNAS* (2000): Vol. 97, no. 7, 3479–3484.

6. August, P, et al. "Hypertension-induced organ damage in african americans: Transforming growth factor-beta excess as a mechanism for increased prevalence." *Current Hypertension Reports* (2007): Vol. 2, no. 2, 184-191.

7. "USRDS 2007 Annual Data Report." www.usrds.org

8. Casimir, J, et al. "[Separation and characterization of N-ethyl-gamma-glutamine from Xerocomus badius.]" *Biochim Biophys Acta* (1960): Vol. 39, 462–468.

9. Kimura, K, et al. "L-Theanine reduces psychological and physiological stress responses." *Biol Psychol* (2007), Vol. 74, no. 1, 39–45.

10. Watanabe, M, et al. "GABA and GABA receptors in the central nervous system and other organs". *Int Rev Cytol* (2002): Vol. 213, 1–47.

11. Tan, X, et al. "Therapeutic role and potential mechanisms of active Vitamin D in renal interstitial fibrosis." *J Steroid Biochem Mol Biol* (2007): Vol. 103, no. 3–5, 491–496.

12. Patel, N. M, et al. "Vitamin D deficiency and anemia in early chronic kidney disease." *Kidney Int* (2010): Vol. 77, no. 8, 715–720.

Chapter 9

1. Allison D. B, et al. "Annual deaths attributable to obesity in the United States." *JAMA* (1999): Vol. 282, no. 16, 1530–1538.

2. Yusuf, S, et al. "Effect of potentially modifiable risk factors associated with myocardial infarction in 52 countries (the INTERHEART study): case-control study." *Lancet* (2004): Vol. 364, no. 9438, 937–952.

3. Peeters, A, et al. "Obesity in adulthood and its consequences for life expectancy: a life-table analysis." *Ann of Intern Med* (2003): Vol. 138, 24–32.

4. McArdle, W. D. *Template: Exercise Physiology, 2nd Edition.* Philadelphia: Lea & Febigier, 1986.

5. Björntorp, P. "Do stress reactions cause abdominal obesity and comorbidities?" *Obesity Reviews* (2001): Vol. 2, no. 2, 73–86.

6. Shintani, M, et al. "Ghrelin, an endogenous growth hormone secretagogue, is a novel Orexigenic peptide that antagonizes Leptin action through the activation of hypothalamic neuropeptide Y/Y1 receptor pathway." *Diabetes* (2001): Vol. 50, 227–232.

7. Heindel, J. J. "Toxicological Highlights. Endocrine Disruptors and the Obesity Epidemic." *Tox Sciences* (2003): Vol. 76, 247–249.

8. Damstra, T, et al. "Global Assessment of the State-of-the-Science of Endocrine Disruptors." *WHO* (2002): no. WHO/PCS/EDC/02.2.

9. Toschke, A. M, et al. "Childhood obesity is associated with maternal smoking in pregnancy." *Eur J Peds* (2002): Vol. 161, 445–448.

10. Levin, E. D. "Animal models of developmental nicotine exposure: possible mechanisms of childhood obesity." *Birth Defects Research, Part B* (2003): Vol. 68, 245.

11. "Body Burden—The Pollution in Newborns. A benchmark investigation of industrial chemicals, pollutants and pesticides in umbilical cord blood." www.ewg.org

12. "Diversity Within African American Communities: Implications for Advancing Research on Weight Issues and Related Disparities." *African American Collaborative Obesity Research Network 3rd Invited Workshop,* 2008.

13. "Obesity, Lifestyles and African Americans—What are the Correlations?" www.imdiversity.com

14. Kremer, R, et al. "Vitamin D Status and its Relationship to Body Fat, Final Height and Peak Bone Mass in Young Women," *Journal of Clinical Endocrinology & Metabolism* (2008): Vol. 94, no. 1, 67–73.

15. McGill, A, et al. "Relationships of low serum vitamin D_3 with anthropometry and markers of the metabolic syndrome and diabetes in overweight and obesity." *Nutrition Journal* (2008): Vol. 7, no. 4.

16. Bray, G. A. "Medical consequences of obesity." *J Clin Endocrinol Metab* (2004): Vol. 89, no. 6, 2583–2589.

17. "Do Diets Work?" www.pbs.org

18. Ibid.

19. "African American Health: African Americans and Diet." www.netwellness.org

20. Boschmann, M, et al. "Water and Thermogenesis." *J of Clinical Endocrine and Metabolism* (2003): Vol. 88, no. 12, 6015–6019.

21. Spiegel, K, et al. "Brief Communication: Sleep Curtailment in Healthy Young Men Is Associated with Decreased Leptin Levels, Elevated Ghrelin Levels, and Increased Hunger and Appetite." *Annals of Internal Medicine* (2004): Vol. 141, no. 11, 846–850.

22. Spiegel, K, et al. "Leptin Levels Are Dependent on Sleep Duration: Relationships with Sympathovagal Balance, Carbohydrate Regulation, Cortisol, and Thyrotropin." *Journal of Clinical Endocrinology and Metabolism* (2004): Vol. 89, no. 11, 5762–5771.

23. Phillips, B. G, et al. "Increases in leptin levels, sympathetic drive, and weight gain in obstructive sleep apnea." *Am J Physiol Heart Circ Physiol* (2000): Vol. 279, no. 1, H234–H237.

24. "Successful Weight Loss with Dieting Is Linked to Vitamin D Levels." www.sciencedaily.com

25. Maki, K. C, et al. "Green tea catechin consumption enhances exercise-induced abdominal fat loss in overweight and obese adults." *The Journal of nutrition* (2009): Vol. 139, no. 2, 264–270. Article

Conclusion

1. "Vitamin D." www.mayoclinic.com

2. Wagner C. L, et al. "Prevention of rickets and vitamin D deficiency in infants, children, and adolescents." *Pediatrics* (2008): Vol. 122, 1142–1152.

3. Colombo, J, et al. "Maternal DHA and the Development of Attention in Infancy and Toddlerhood." *Child Development* (2004): Vol. 75, no. 4, 1254–1267.

4. Helland, I. B, et al. "Maternal supplementation with very-long-chain n-3 fatty acids during pregnancy and lactation augments children's IQ at 4 years of age." *Pediatrics* (2003): Vol. 111, no. 1, 39–44.

5. Cohen, J. T, et al. "A quantitative analysis of prenatal intake of n-3 polyunsaturated fatty acids and cognitive development." *Am J Prev Med* (2005): Vol. 29, no. 4, 366–374.

6. Daniels, J. L, et al. "Fish intake during pregnancy and early cognitive development of offspring." *Epidemiology* (2004): Vol. 15, no. 4, 394–402.

7. Cheruku, S. R, et al. "Higher maternal plasma docosahexaenoic acid during pregnancy is associated with more mature neonatal sleep-state patterning." *Am J Clin Nutr* (2002): Vol. 76, no. 3, 608–613.

8. Borja-Hart, N. L. and Marin, J. "Role of omega-3 fatty acids for prevention or treatment of perinatal depression." *Pharmacotherapy* (2010): Vol. 30, no. 2, 210–216.

9. FDA 1990–2004. "National Marine Fisheries Service Survey of Trace Elements in the Fishery Resource" Report 1978.

10. "Facts about Folate." www.eatrightontario.ca

11. "Complementary and Alternative Medicine: Flaxseed and Flaxseed Oil." www.intelihealth.com

12. Shaw, G. M, et al. "Periconceptional vitamin use, dietary folate, and the occurrence of neural tube defects." *Epidemiology* (1995): Vol. 6, no. 3, 219–226.

13. Wilcox A. J, et al. "Folic acid supplements and risk of facial clefts: national population based case-control study." *BMJ* (2007): Vol. 334, no. 7591, 464.

14. Goh, Y. I. and Koren, G. "Folic acid in pregnancy and fetal outcomes." *J Obstet Gynaecol* (2008): Vol. 28, no. 3, 3–13.

15. "Folic Acid: What Should You Know?" www.cdc.gov

About the Author

Richard W. Walker, Jr., MD, was born in New York City and raised in the Johnson Projects of Spanish Harlem. As a child, he suffered from many different medical conditions, including pneumonia, appendicitis, heart murmurs, and more. From his frequent visits to his "favorite" hospital, Columbia Presbyterian in Washington Heights, he still recalls the image of black stethoscopes against all-white uniforms. It was through these experiences that his desire to become a physician was born.

By the time he was in high school, however, his goal was simply to graduate. His tough neighborhood, the discouragement of school counselors, and an undiagnosed case of dyslexia all made him see himself as "not college material," despite his notably high I.Q. After barely squeaking by, he received his high school diploma only to drop out of community college due to poor grades. Seeking direction, he chose to join the Armed Forces. It was during this time that he met the person who would change his life, his future wife, Marvia. The two were married after dating for only three months.

Thanks to his success as a member of the United States Air Force, and Marvia's persistence and inspiration, he decided to give college another try. He began taking courses one at a time and performed very well in all of them. By the time he was honorably discharged from the Air Force, he had a full semester's credits behind him. In 1969, he enrolled at John Jay College of

Criminal Justice in New York City, graduating with a bachelor's degree in forensic science in 1971, all while working a full-time job and supporting a family of four. While studying for a master's degree at the same institution, he was approached by Professor Alexander Joseph, PhD, the Dean of the science department, who had learned of the training the promising student had received as a combat medic in the Armed Forces. Recognizing his potential, Dr. Joseph strongly encouraged him to go to medical school. With very little money and lots of bills to pay, Richard initially balked at the suggestion. But after considerable persuasion, he reluctantly agreed to follow Dr. Joseph's advice. Before long, he was accepting his medical degree from the Albert Einstein College of Medicine and moving on to a residency program in obstetrics and gynecology at the University of Michigan.

Upon completion of his residency in 1978, Dr. Walker relocated to Houston, Texas to begin his medical practice. Since then, he has changed his focus to integrative medicine, also known as orthomolecular medicine, in hopes of curing or preventing disease instead of merely managing it. This growing field integrates the best of traditional and alternative medical thought. He has also expanded into the fields of age management (anti-aging) and environmental medicine in his search for all possible approaches to therapy. According to the author, "people deserve the best there is available in healthcare."

Dr. Walker has served on the faculty of the University of Texas Medical Center, and is the founder and medical director of HEALTHe & WELL, PC, a Houston-based health center. In addition to being a published writer, he is a highly sought-after speaker. The author attributes his remarkable and unlikely success to his wife, Marvia, who was the voice of encouragement and the force behind his achievement; his children, who, although they did not know the depth of his struggle, always said, "Dad, you can do it;" Professor Joseph, who saw something in him that he didn't know was there; and Major Ray Sumners, who was a guiding light to him throughout his time in the Air Force and the person who taught him how to succeed.

Index

The Square One Health Guides

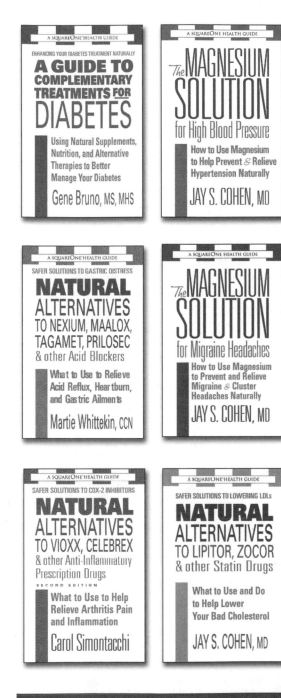

Written by health professionals, these concise, easy-to-read books focus on a wide range of important health concerns. From migraine headaches to high cholesterol, each title looks at a specific problem; each provides a clear explanation of the disorder, its causes, and its symptoms; and each offers natural solutions that can either greatly reduce or completely eliminate the problem.

A Guide to Complementary Treatments for Diabetes
$7.95 US • 240 pages • ISBN 978-0-7570-0322-6

The Magnesium Solution for High Blood Pressure
$5.95 US • 96 pages • ISBN 978-0-7570-0255-7

Natural Alternatives to Nexium, Maalox, Tagamet, Prilosec & Other Acid Blockers
$7.95 US • 272 pages • ISBN 978-0-7570-0210-6

The Magnesium Solution for Migraine Headaches
$5.95 US • 96 pages • ISBN 978-0-7570-0256-4

Natural Alternatives to Vioxx, Celebrex & Other Anti-Inflammatory Prescription Drugs, SECOND EDITION
$5.95 US • 128 pages • ISBN 978-0-7570-0278-6

Natural Alternatives to Lipitor, Zocor & Other Statin Drugs
$7.95 US • 144 pages • ISBN 978-0-7570-0286-1

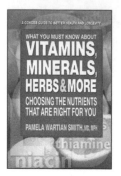
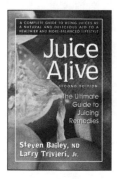